super easy

Diabetic Diet

Cookbook after 50

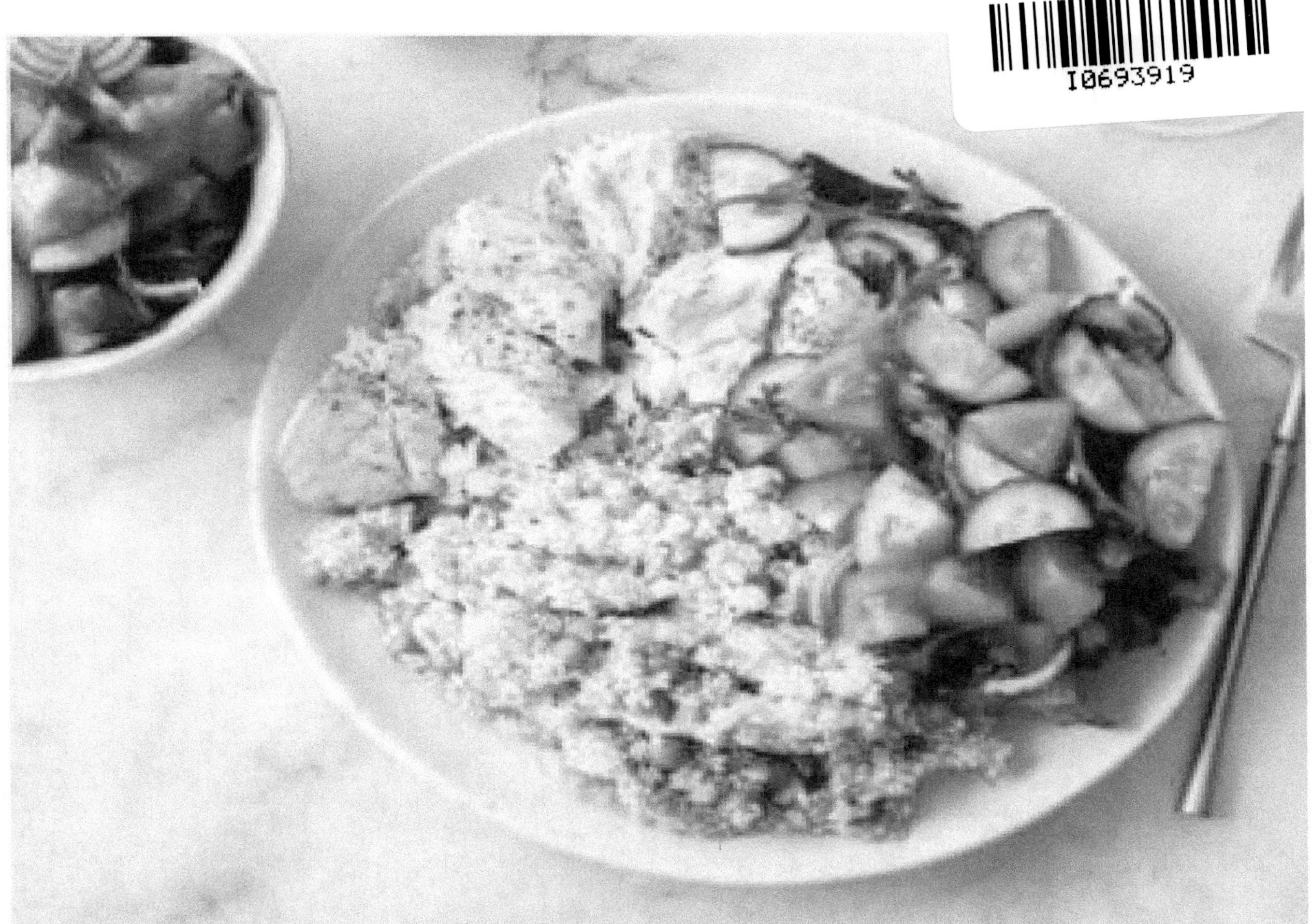

The Ultimate Complete Guide to 2000 Days of Delicious Low Carb Low Sugar Easy-to-Make Recipes in Less Than 30 Minutes for Prediabetes & Type 2 Diabetes for Longevity and Wellbeing + Meal Plan

Jessica C. James

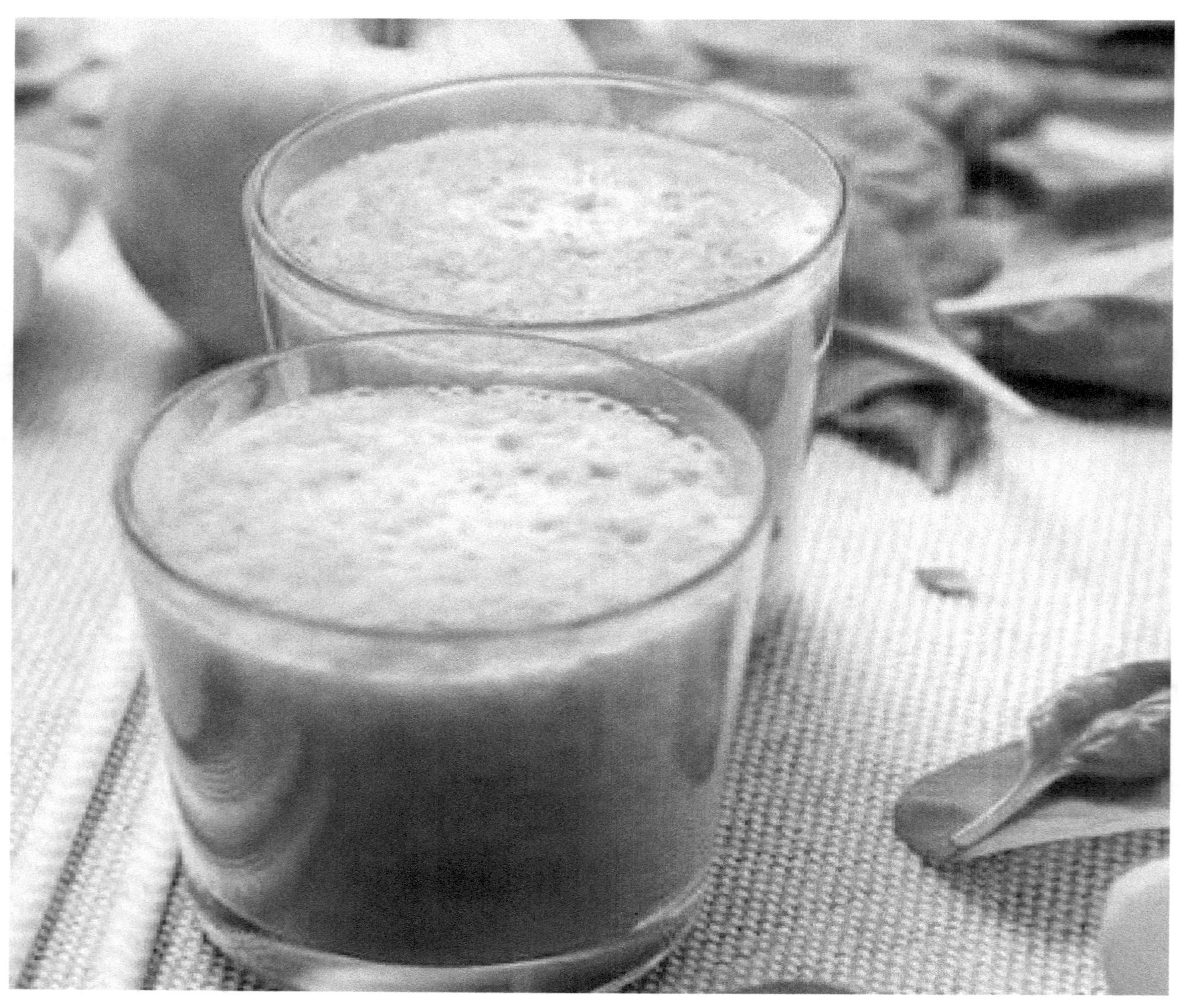

Welcome!

We're thrilled you chose "Super Easy Diabetic Diet Cookbook After 50." This book is your perfect companion for managing diabetes with delicious, fuss-free recipes designed just for you. Discover 100+ easy meals with juicing for diabetics, a stress-free meal plan, and a guide to smart food choices all to empower you for a healthy, flavorful future! Thank you for selecting our book to accompany you on your health journey.

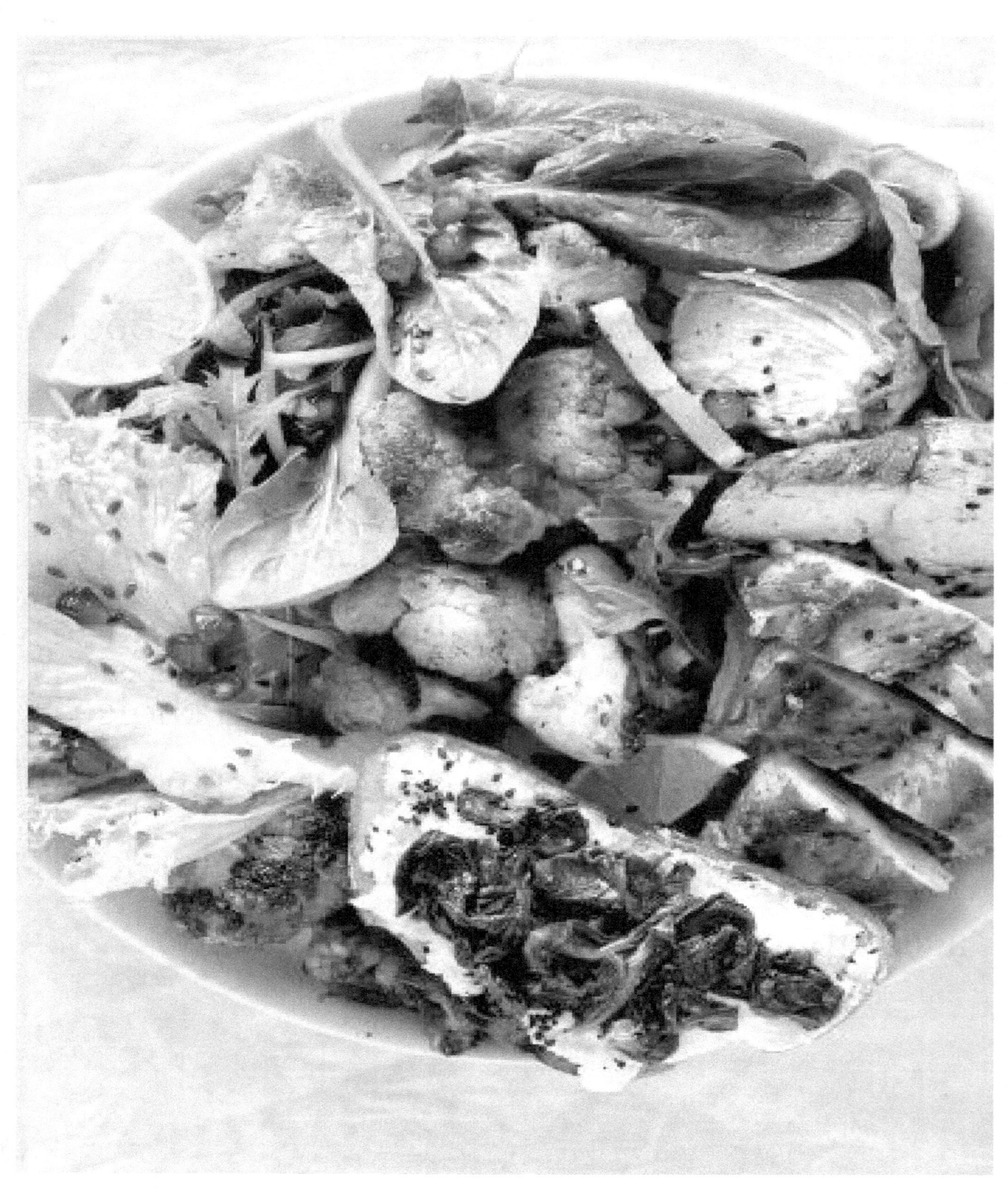

TABLE OF CONTENT

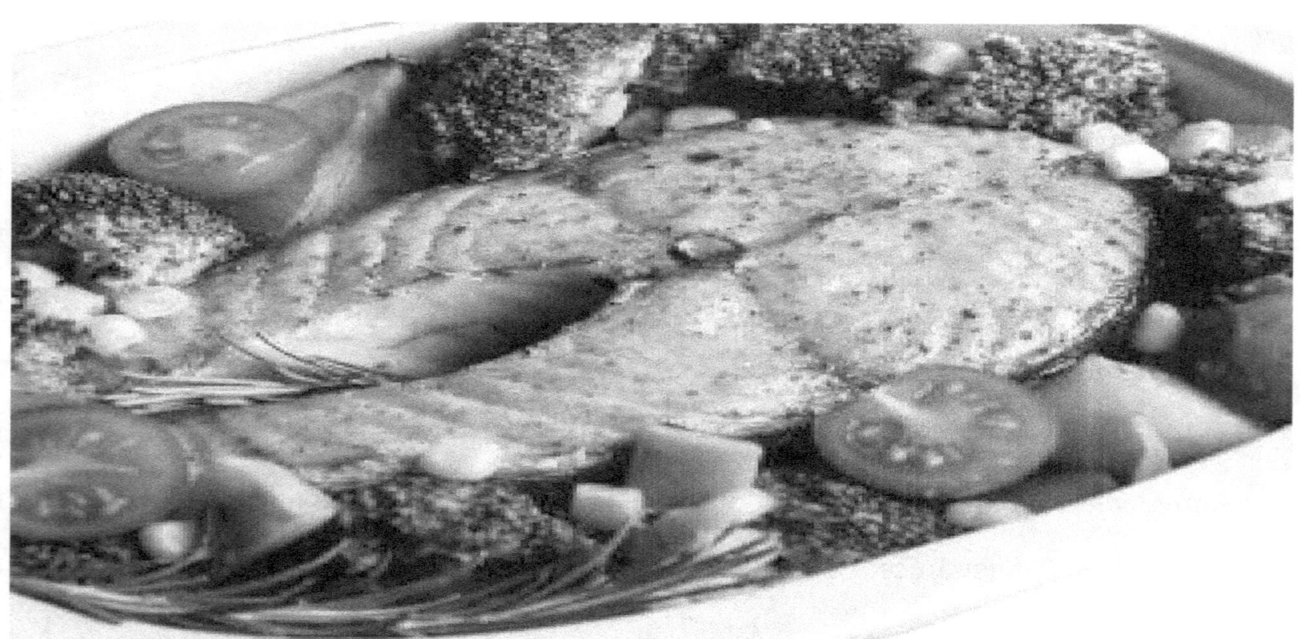

INTRODUCTION

In our modern world, where convenience often trumps health, the prevalence of diabetes has become a significant concern. It's a condition that affects millions of lives worldwide, touching the young and old alike. Diabetes, particularly Type 2 diabetes, has emerged as a silent epidemic, silently creeping into our lives and altering the way we approach food, health, and well-being.

The statistics are staggering: approximately 37.3 million people in the United States alone grapple with diabetes, accounting for about 11% of the population. What's even more concerning is that Type 2 diabetes, the most common form, makes up 90% to 95% of all diabetes cases. These numbers paint a stark reality, one that underscores the urgent need for proactive measures to address this growing health crisis.

Beyond the borders of any single nation, diabetes casts a global shadow. A staggering 537 million adults worldwide live with diabetes, a number projected to skyrocket to 643 million by 2030 and a daunting 783 million by 2045. These figures not only illustrate the scale of the challenge we face but also serve as a sobering reminder of the imperative to take action.

Yet, behind these statistics lie stories—stories of resilience, determination, and hope. Each number represents a person, a family, a community grappling with the daily realities of diabetes.

It's a condition that impacts every aspect of life, from mealtime choices to long-term health outcomes, from emotional well-being to financial stability.

In the face of such daunting numbers and personal challenges, it's easy to feel overwhelmed and disheartened. But amidst the darkness, there is a beacon of hope—a glimmer of light shining through the clouds. That beacon is the Super Easy Diabetic Diet Cookbook.

This cookbook is more than just a collection of recipes; it's a lifeline for those navigating the complex landscape of diabetes management. It's a testament to the power of food as medicine, as nourishment for both body and soul.

With its carefully curated selection of diabetic-friendly recipes, this cookbook empowers individuals to take control of their health and well-being, one delicious meal at a time.

But the Super Easy Diabetic Diet Cookbook is not just about what's on the plate; it's about what's in the heart. It's about fostering a sense of community, solidarity, and support among those facing similar challenges. It's about reminding each other that we're not alone on this journey—that together, we can overcome obstacles and embrace a healthier, happier future.

So, as you embark on this culinary adventure, remember that you're not just cooking a meal; you're nourishing your body, nurturing your spirit, and reclaiming your health. Let the Super Easy Diabetic Diet Cookbook be your guide, your companion, and your source of inspiration on this journey toward wellness. Together, let's turn the tide against diabetes and embrace a flavorful, balanced lifestyle that celebrates the joys of food and the gift of good health.

CHAPTER 1

What is Diabetes?

Diabetes is a condition that affects how your body uses glucose, which is a type of sugar and a crucial source of energy for your cells. When you eat food, your body breaks down carbohydrates into glucose, which then enters your bloodstream.

Normally, the hormone insulin, produced by the pancreas, helps glucose enter your cells to be used for energy. However, in diabetes, there's a problem with insulin production or how your body uses insulin, leading to high levels of glucose in your blood.

Types of Diabetes:

Type 1 Diabetes

Type 1 diabetes is a chronic condition where the immune system mistakenly attacks the insulin-producing cells in the pancreas. These cells, called beta cells, are responsible for producing insulin, a hormone crucial for regulating blood sugar levels. Without enough insulin, glucose cannot enter the body's cells to provide energy, leading to high levels of sugar in the bloodstream.

Key Points:

Autoimmune Response: In Type 1 diabetes, the body's immune system mistakenly identifies the beta cells as foreign invaders and destroys them. The exact cause of this autoimmune response is not fully understood, but genetic and environmental factors likely play a role.

Onset and Diagnosis: Type 1 diabetes often develops in childhood or adolescence, although it can occur at any age. Symptoms typically appear suddenly and include excessive thirst, frequent urination, weight loss, fatigue, and blurred vision. Blood tests measuring glucose levels and other markers are used to diagnose the condition.

Treatment: People with Type 1 diabetes require lifelong insulin therapy to replace the insulin their pancreas no longer produces. Insulin can be administered through injections or an insulin pump. The goal of treatment is to maintain blood sugar levels within a target range to prevent complications.

Blood Sugar Monitoring: Regular monitoring of blood sugar levels is essential for managing Type 1 diabetes. This involves using a glucose meter to measure blood sugar levels throughout the day, especially before and after meals, exercise, and sleep.

Meal Planning: Consistent carbohydrate intake and balanced nutrition are important for managing blood sugar levels. Meal planning may involve counting carbohydrates, monitoring portion sizes, and choosing foods that have a minimal impact on blood sugar.

Physical Activity: Exercise can help regulate blood sugar levels by increasing insulin sensitivity and promoting glucose uptake by muscles. However, individuals with Type 1 diabetes may need to adjust their insulin doses or carbohydrate intake to prevent blood sugar fluctuations during exercise.

Complications: Poorly controlled Type 1 diabetes can lead to serious complications over time, including heart disease, kidney damage, nerve damage, vision problems, and circulation issues. Regular medical check-ups and adherence to treatment are crucial for minimizing the risk of complications.

Type 2 Diabetes

Type 2 diabetes is a chronic condition characterized by insulin resistance, where the body's cells become resistant to the effects of insulin, or insufficient insulin production by the pancreas. This results in elevated blood sugar levels, known as hyperglycemia. Type 2 diabetes is the most common form of diabetes, typically occurring in adults, but it can also develop in children and adolescents.

Key Points:

Insulin Resistance: In Type 2 diabetes, the body's cells become resistant to insulin, preventing glucose from entering the cells effectively. Initially, the pancreas compensates by producing more insulin, but over time, it may not be able to keep up with the increased demand, leading to elevated blood sugar levels.

Risk Factors: Several factors increase the risk of developing Type 2 diabetes, including obesity, sedentary lifestyle, unhealthy diet, family history of diabetes, age (particularly over 45), ethnicity (African American, Hispanic/Latino, Native American, Asian American, Pacific Islander), and gestational diabetes during pregnancy.

Symptoms: Symptoms of Type 2 diabetes may develop gradually and include increased thirst, frequent urination, fatigue, blurred vision, slow healing of wounds, and tingling or numbness in the hands or feet. Many individuals may have no symptoms or only mild symptoms, leading to delayed diagnosis.

Diagnosis: Diagnosis of Type 2 diabetes is typically based on blood tests measuring fasting blood glucose levels, oral glucose tolerance test (OGTT), or HbA1c levels (average blood sugar levels over the past 2-3 months). Screening for diabetes is recommended for individuals with risk factors or symptoms.

Treatment: Treatment for Type 2 diabetes aims to manage blood sugar levels and prevent complications. Lifestyle modifications, including healthy eating, regular physical activity, and weight management, are foundational. Medications such as oral antidiabetic drugs (e.g., metformin, sulfonylureas, DPP-4 inhibitors) or injectable insulin may be prescribed to lower blood sugar levels when lifestyle changes alone are insufficient.

Blood Sugar Monitoring: Regular monitoring of blood sugar levels is important for individuals with Type 2 diabetes to assess the effectiveness of treatment and make adjustments as needed. Self-monitoring using a glucose meter helps track blood sugar levels and identify patterns over time.

Complications: Poorly controlled Type 2 diabetes can lead to serious complications, including heart disease, stroke, kidney disease, nerve damage (neuropathy), vision problems (retinopathy), foot problems, and skin conditions. Comprehensive diabetes management, including regular medical check-ups and screenings, is essential for preventing or delaying complications.

Prevention: Lifestyle modifications, such as maintaining a healthy weight, eating a balanced diet, engaging in regular physical activity, and avoiding tobacco use, can help prevent or delay the onset of Type 2 diabetes, especially in individuals at high risk.

While Type 2 diabetes requires lifelong management, early diagnosis, proper treatment, and lifestyle changes can help individuals effectively control their blood sugar levels and reduce the risk of complications, improving overall health and well-being.

Gestational Diabetes

Gestational diabetes is a type of diabetes that develops during pregnancy. It occurs when the body cannot produce enough insulin to meet the increased demands of pregnancy, leading to elevated blood sugar levels. Gestational diabetes usually develops around the 24th to 28th week of pregnancy and typically resolves after childbirth. However, it requires careful management to prevent complications for both the mother and the baby.

Key Points:

Risk Factors: While any pregnant woman can develop gestational diabetes, certain factors increase the risk, including being overweight or obese, having a family history of diabetes, being older than 25, previously giving birth to a baby weighing over 9 pounds, and belonging to certain ethnic groups (such as African American, Hispanic/Latino, Native American, Asian American, or Pacific Islander).

Cause: During pregnancy, the placenta produces hormones that help the baby grow but can also interfere with the body's insulin action, leading to insulin resistance. If the pancreas cannot produce enough insulin to overcome this resistance, blood sugar levels rise, resulting in gestational diabetes.

Screening and Diagnosis: Screening for gestational diabetes typically occurs between the 24th and 28th weeks of pregnancy. It involves a glucose challenge test

(GCT), followed by a glucose tolerance test (GTT) if the GCT results are abnormal. Diagnosis is made when blood sugar levels are higher than normal but not yet at the diabetes level.

Complications: Gestational diabetes increases the risk of complications for both the mother and the baby. For the mother, it can lead to preeclampsia (high blood pressure during pregnancy), cesarean delivery, and an increased risk of developing Type 2 diabetes later in life. For the baby, complications may include macrosomia (large birth weight), birth injuries, hypoglycemia (low blood sugar) after birth, and an increased risk of developing obesity and Type 2 diabetes later in life.

Management: Treatment for gestational diabetes focuses on controlling blood sugar levels to reduce the risk of complications. This typically involves lifestyle modifications, such as following a healthy diet, monitoring blood sugar levels regularly, engaging in regular physical activity (under the guidance of a healthcare provider), and sometimes insulin therapy or oral medication if blood sugar levels remain high despite lifestyle changes.

Postpartum Follow-up: After childbirth, women who had gestational diabetes should undergo postpartum screening to evaluate their blood sugar levels. They are also at increased risk of developing Type 2 diabetes in the future and should undergo regular screening for diabetes during follow-up visits with their healthcare provider.

Prevention: While gestational diabetes cannot always be prevented, maintaining a healthy lifestyle before and during pregnancy can help reduce the risk. This includes achieving a healthy weight before pregnancy, eating a balanced diet, engaging in regular physical activity, and attending prenatal care appointments.

Prediabetes is a condition where blood sugar levels are higher than normal but not yet high enough to be diagnosed as Type 2 diabetes.

It serves as a warning sign that individuals are at increased risk of developing Type 2 diabetes if preventive measures are not taken.

Key Points:

Risk Factors: Several factors increase the risk of developing prediabetes, including being overweight or obese, lack of physical activity, unhealthy diet, family history of diabetes, age (particularly over 45), ethnicity (African American, Hispanic/Latino, Native American, Asian American, Pacific Islander), and history of gestational diabetes or polycystic ovary syndrome (PCOS).

Importance of Diagnosis: Identifying prediabetes is crucial as it provides an opportunity for early intervention to prevent or delay the progression to Type 2 diabetes. Many individuals with prediabetes may have no symptoms or only mild symptoms, making diagnosis through blood tests essential.

Reversibility: The good news is that prediabetes can often be reversed through lifestyle changes, such as adopting a healthy diet, increasing physical activity, and losing weight if overweight or obese. Research has shown that losing even a modest amount of weight (5-7% of body weight) and engaging in regular physical activity (at least 150 minutes per week) can significantly reduce the risk of developing Type 2 diabetes.

Type 3c Diabetes: This form of diabetes occurs when the pancreas experiences damage that affects its ability to produce insulin. The damage to the pancreas can result from conditions such as pancreatitis (inflammation of the pancreas), pancreatic cancer, cystic fibrosis (a genetic disorder affecting the lungs and digestive system), or hemochromatosis (a condition where iron accumulates in the body). Type 3c diabetes is relatively rare compared to other types of diabetes.

Latent Autoimmune Diabetes in Adults (LADA): LADA is a type of diabetes that shares features of both Type 1 and Type 2 diabetes. Like Type 1 diabetes, LADA is characterized by autoimmune destruction of the insulin-producing beta cells in the pancreas. However, unlike Type 1 diabetes, LADA typically develops more slowly and is diagnosed in adults, often after the age of 30. Individuals with LADA may initially be misdiagnosed as having Type 2 diabetes due to their older age at diagnosis and the gradual onset of symptoms.

Maturity-Onset Diabetes of the Young (MODY): MODY is a rare form of diabetes caused by mutations in specific genes that affect how the pancreas produces insulin. It is often inherited in an autosomal dominant pattern, meaning that a person only needs to inherit one copy of the mutated gene from either parent to develop the condition. MODY typically manifests before the age of 25 and accounts for about 1-5% of all diabetes cases. There are several subtypes of MODY, each caused by mutations in different genes, and each subtype may have distinct clinical features and treatment implications.

Neonatal Diabetes: Neonatal diabetes is a rare form of diabetes that occurs in infants under six months of age.

It is usually caused by genetic mutations that affect insulin production or function. Neonatal diabetes can be either transient, where the condition resolves within the first few months of life but may recur later in life, or permanent, where the condition persists throughout life. Genetic testing is often used to diagnose neonatal diabetes and guide treatment decisions.

Brittle Diabetes: Brittle diabetes, also known as labile diabetes or unstable diabetes, is a term used to describe a severe form of Type 1 diabetes characterized by unpredictable and frequent fluctuations in blood sugar levels, leading to episodes of hyperglycemia (high blood sugar) and hypoglycemia (low blood sugar).

Individuals with brittle diabetes often struggle to maintain stable blood sugar control despite rigorous management efforts, and they may be at increased risk of diabetes-related complications. Management of brittle diabetes may require intensive insulin therapy, continuous glucose monitoring, and close medical supervision.

symptoms of diabetics

Symptoms of diabetes can vary depending on the type of diabetes and the individual. Here are the common symptoms associated with diabetes:

Frequent Urination (Polyuria): Excess sugar in the blood can cause the kidneys to work harder to filter and absorb the sugar, leading to increased urination.

Increased Thirst (Polydipsia): Excessive urination can lead to dehydration, triggering thirst to replenish lost fluids.

Extreme Hunger (Polyphagia): Despite eating regularly, individuals with diabetes may experience persistent hunger due to the body's inability to properly utilize glucose for energy.

Unexplained Weight Loss: In Type 1 diabetes, the body may break down muscle and fat tissue for energy due to the absence of insulin. In Type 2 diabetes, inadequate insulin action can prevent glucose from entering cells, leading to weight loss.

Fatigue: Feeling tired or lethargic is common in diabetes, as the body's cells may not receive enough glucose for energy production.

Blurred Vision: High blood sugar levels can cause changes in the shape of the lens of the eye, resulting in blurry or distorted vision.

Slow Healing of Wounds: Diabetes can impair the body's ability to heal wounds and injuries due to poor circulation and compromised immune function.

Frequent Infections: High blood sugar levels can weaken the immune system, making individuals with diabetes more susceptible to infections, such as urinary tract infections, yeast infections, and skin infections.

Tingling or Numbness in Hands and Feet (Peripheral Neuropathy): Diabetes can damage nerves, leading to tingling, numbness, or pain, particularly in the hands and feet.

Dry Skin: Diabetes can cause dehydration, leading to dry, itchy skin. Poor circulation and nerve damage can also contribute to skin problems.

Yeast Infections (Genital Itching or Thrush): Women with diabetes may experience frequent yeast infections, while both men and women may develop thrush, a fungal infection in the mouth or throat.

Increased Risk of Cardiovascular Symptoms: Diabetes significantly increases the risk of cardiovascular complications, such as chest pain (angina), heart attack, and stroke. Symptoms may include chest discomfort, shortness of breath, and palpitations.

Insulin Resistance: In Type 2 diabetes, insulin resistance plays a central role.

This occurs when cells in the muscles, fat, and liver fail to respond adequately to insulin. Factors contributing to insulin resistance include obesity, sedentary lifestyle, unhealthy diet, hormonal imbalances, genetic predisposition, and certain medications.

Autoimmune Disease: Type 1 diabetes and Latent Autoimmune Diabetes in Adults (LADA) result from an autoimmune response in which the body's immune system mistakenly attacks and destroys the insulin-producing beta cells in the pancreas. The exact triggers for this autoimmune reaction are not fully understood, but genetic predisposition and environmental factors likely play a role.

Hormonal Imbalances: Gestational diabetes can develop during pregnancy due to hormonal changes that lead to insulin resistance.

The placenta produces hormones that can interfere with insulin action, particularly in women with pre-existing risk factors. Other hormone-related conditions, such as acromegaly and Cushing syndrome, can also contribute to insulin resistance and Type 2 diabetes.

Pancreatic Damage: Damage to the pancreas from conditions like pancreatitis, pancreatic surgery, or injury can impair its ability to produce insulin, leading to Type 3c diabetes. This form of diabetes is relatively rare but underscores the importance of pancreatic function in glucose regulation.

Genetic Mutations: Certain genetic mutations can predispose individuals to specific types of diabetes. Maturity-Onset Diabetes of the Young (MODY) and neonatal diabetes are examples of monogenic forms of diabetes caused by genetic defects that affect insulin production or function.

Medications: Long-term use of certain medications can increase the risk of developing Type 2 diabetes. Examples include medications for HIV/AIDS treatment and corticosteroids used to manage conditions like asthma, rheumatoid arthritis, and autoimmune diseases. These medications can interfere with insulin sensitivity or impair pancreatic function over time.

Understanding the underlying causes of diabetes is essential for developing targeted interventions and treatment strategies. Lifestyle modifications, including healthy eating, regular physical activity, weight management, and medication management, are crucial components of diabetes management regardless of the underlying cause. Additionally, early detection through screening and regular medical check-ups can help identify and manage diabetes effectively.

Complications of Diabetes

Diabetes can lead to a range of acute and long-term complications, primarily due to prolonged high blood sugar levels. These complications can affect various organs and systems in the body, posing significant health risks. Here's an overview of the complications associated with diabetes:

Hyperosmolar Hyperglycemic State (HHS): Mainly affecting individuals with Type 2 diabetes, HHS occurs when blood sugar levels become extremely high (over 600 mg/dL) for an extended period. It can result in severe dehydration, confusion, and requires immediate medical intervention.

Diabetic Ketoacidosis (DKA): Predominantly seen in individuals with Type 1 diabetes or undiagnosed Type 1 diabetes, DKA occurs when the body lacks sufficient insulin to utilize glucose for energy, leading to the breakdown of fat and the production of acidic ketones.

Symptoms include labored breathing, vomiting, and loss of consciousness, necessitating immediate medical treatment.

Severe Hypoglycemia: Hypoglycemia, or low blood sugar, can be life-threatening when levels drop below a healthy range, particularly in individuals using insulin. Severe hypoglycemia can cause blurred vision, disorientation, seizures, and requires emergency intervention with glucagon or medical assistance.

Long-Term Diabetes Complications:

Cardiovascular Issues: Diabetes significantly increases the risk of cardiovascular diseases, including coronary artery disease, heart attack, stroke, and atherosclerosis, due to damage to blood vessels and increased susceptibility to plaque buildup.

Nerve Damage (Neuropathy): Elevated blood sugar levels can damage nerves, leading to symptoms such as numbness, tingling, or pain, particularly in the hands and feet.

Nephropathy: Diabetes-related kidney damage can progress to kidney failure, necessitating dialysis or transplant.

Retinopathy: Damage to the blood vessels in the retina can cause vision impairment or blindness.

Diabetes-Related Foot Conditions: Nerve damage and poor circulation increase the risk of foot ulcers, infections, and the need for amputations.

Skin Infections: Elevated blood sugar levels create a favorable environment for infections, leading to skin complications.

Sexual Dysfunction: Diabetes-related nerve and blood vessel damage can cause sexual dysfunction, such as erectile dysfunction or vaginal dryness.

Gastroparesis: Delayed stomach emptying can lead to gastrointestinal symptoms, such as nausea, vomiting, and difficulty digesting food.

Hearing Loss: Diabetes is associated with an increased risk of hearing impairment.

Oral Health Issues: Gum disease (periodontal disease) and other oral health problems are more common in individuals with diabetes.

Preventing Diabetes

While some forms of diabetes, such as autoimmune and genetic types, cannot be prevented, there are steps you can take to lower your risk of developing prediabetes, Type 2 diabetes, and gestational diabetes. Here are some preventive measures you can incorporate into your lifestyle:

Healthy Diet: Follow a balanced and nutritious diet, such as the Mediterranean diet, rich in fruits, vegetables, whole grains, lean proteins, and healthy fats. Limit processed foods, sugary snacks, and beverages high in added sugars.

Regular Physical Activity: Aim for at least 30 minutes of moderate-intensity exercise on most days of the week. Choose activities you enjoy, such as walking, cycling, swimming, or dancing, to make exercise a regular part of your routine.

Maintain a Healthy Weight: Work towards achieving and maintaining a weight that is appropriate for your height and body type. Even modest weight loss can significantly reduce the risk of developing Type 2 diabetes.

Stress Management: Find healthy ways to cope with stress, such as relaxation techniques, mindfulness meditation, yoga, or engaging in hobbies and activities you enjoy.

Limit Alcohol Consumption: If you choose to drink alcohol, do so in moderation. Limit intake to no more than one drink per day for women and up to two drinks per day for men.

Prioritize Sleep: Aim for 7 to 9 hours of quality sleep each night. Address any sleep disorders, such as sleep apnea, through appropriate treatment.

Quit Smoking: If you smoke, seek support and resources to quit smoking. Smoking increases the risk of developing Type 2 diabetes and exacerbates complications associated with the disease.

Medication Management: If you have existing risk factors for heart disease, such as high blood pressure or high cholesterol, take medications as directed by your healthcare provider to manage these conditions effectively.

Management and Treatment of Diabetes

Managing diabetes involves a comprehensive approach tailored to individual needs and circumstances. While diabetes management strategies may vary, they generally encompass four main aspects:

Blood Sugar Monitoring: Regular monitoring of blood sugar (glucose) levels is crucial for assessing the effectiveness of treatment plans and making necessary adjustments.

This may involve frequent checks using a glucose meter and finger stick, or continuous glucose monitoring (CGM) systems. Collaborating with healthcare providers helps establish target blood sugar ranges suitable for each individual.

Medications:

Oral Diabetes Medications: These medications are taken by mouth and are primarily used to manage blood sugar levels in individuals with Type 2 diabetes or prediabetes.

Common oral medications, such as metformin, assist in regulating blood sugar levels.

Insulin Therapy: Individuals with Type 1 diabetes require synthetic insulin injections to maintain blood sugar control. Some people with Type 2 diabetes may also need insulin therapy, which can be administered via various methods, including syringe injections, insulin pens, insulin pumps, or rapid-acting inhaled insulin. Insulin types vary in onset, duration, and speed of action, allowing for customized treatment plans.

Dietary Management: Adopting a healthy diet is essential for managing diabetes effectively. Meal planning, carbohydrate counting, and selecting nutritious foods help regulate blood sugar levels. For individuals on insulin therapy, coordinating carbohydrate intake with insulin doses is crucial to maintain glycemic control. A balanced diet supports weight management and reduces the risk of heart disease.

Physical Activity: Regular exercise plays a vital role in diabetes management by improving insulin sensitivity and reducing insulin resistance.

Engaging in physical activity helps control blood sugar levels, promotes weight loss or maintenance, and enhances overall cardiovascular health. Incorporating aerobic exercises, strength training, and flexibility exercises into daily routines is beneficial for all individuals with diabetes.

In addition to these core management strategies, individuals with diabetes should prioritize maintaining a healthy weight, managing blood pressure and cholesterol levels, and addressing any other risk factors for heart disease. Multidisciplinary collaboration involving healthcare providers, dietitians, diabetes educators, and other specialists supports comprehensive diabetes care.

Managing Blood Sugar Levels

Managing blood sugar levels is a cornerstone of diabetes management and involves various strategies to keep glucose levels within a healthy range. Here's an overview of effective ways to manage blood sugar levels:

Blood Sugar Monitoring: Regularly checking blood sugar levels using a glucose meter or continuous glucose monitoring (CGM) system helps track fluctuations and informs treatment decisions. Monitoring frequency may vary based on individual needs and treatment plans.

Medication Adherence: Taking prescribed diabetes medications, such as insulin or oral medications, as directed by healthcare providers is crucial for regulating blood sugar levels. Adhering to medication schedules helps maintain consistent glucose control.

Healthy Eating Habits:

Carbohydrate Management: Monitoring carbohydrate intake and distributing it evenly throughout meals can help manage blood sugar levels.

Carbohydrate counting and glycemic index awareness assist in selecting foods that have minimal impact on blood sugar.

Balanced Diet: Emphasizing whole foods, including fruits, vegetables, lean proteins, and whole grains, supports stable blood sugar levels. Portion control, meal timing, and moderation of high-sugar or high-fat foods contribute to balanced eating habits.

Physical Activity: Incorporating regular exercise into daily routines improves insulin sensitivity and helps lower blood sugar levels. Engaging in aerobic activities, strength training, or flexibility exercises for at least 150 minutes per week promotes glucose utilization and overall health.

Stress Management: Practicing stress-reducing techniques, such as mindfulness, meditation, deep breathing exercises, or hobbies, helps mitigate stress-related spikes in blood sugar levels.

Hydration: Drinking an adequate amount of water throughout the day supports kidney function and helps prevent dehydration, which can affect blood sugar levels.

Medication Adjustments: Collaborating with healthcare providers to adjust medication dosages or treatment plans based on blood sugar monitoring results, lifestyle changes, or other factors optimizes glucose control.

Regular Healthcare Visits: Attending regular check-ups with healthcare providers allows for ongoing assessment of blood sugar levels, monitoring of diabetes-related complications, and adjustment of management strategies as needed.

Sleep Hygiene: Prioritizing quality sleep and establishing consistent sleep patterns promote hormonal balance and help regulate blood sugar levels. Aim for 7 to 9 hours of uninterrupted sleep per night.

Education and Support: Participating in diabetes education programs, support groups, or counseling sessions provides valuable information, resources, and emotional support for managing blood sugar levels effectively.

Your blood sugar target represents the range you aim to achieve as consistently as possible. It's crucial to maintain blood sugar levels within this target range to prevent or delay serious long-term health issues like heart disease, vision impairment, and kidney disease. Keeping your blood sugar within range can also boost your energy levels and mood.

How can I check my blood sugar?

You can check your blood sugar using a blood sugar meter (glucometer) or a continuous glucose monitor (CGM). A blood sugar meter measures glucose levels in a small blood sample, typically obtained from your fingertip. A CGM employs a sensor placed under the skin to monitor blood sugar levels continuously. If you use a CGM, it's still essential to conduct daily checks with a blood sugar meter to ensure accuracy.

When should I check my blood sugar?

The frequency of blood sugar checks depends on your diabetes type and medication regimen. Typical times to check blood sugar include upon waking up, before meals, two hours after meals, and at bedtime. If you have Type 1 diabetes, use insulin, or experience frequent low blood sugar.

What are blood sugar targets?

Blood sugar targets refer to the desired range you aim to maintain. Typical targets include:

Before meals: 80 to 130 mg/dL

Two hours after meals: Less than 180 mg/dL

Your specific targets may vary based on factors like age, existing health conditions, and individual circumstances. Discuss with your healthcare team to determine the best targets for you.

What causes low blood sugar?

Low blood sugar (hypoglycemia) can result from various factors, including skipped meals, excessive insulin doses, certain medications, increased physical activity, and alcohol consumption. Symptoms vary among individuals but may include shaking, sweating, nervousness, confusion, dizziness, and hunger. Recognizing your unique symptoms is crucial for early detection and treatment.

How can I treat low blood sugar?

If your blood sugar drops below 70 mg/dL, take immediate action by consuming glucose tablets, fruit juice, regular soda, or hard candy to raise your blood sugar levels. Wait 15 minutes, then recheck your blood sugar and repeat treatment if necessary. If you experience hypoglycemia unawareness, monitor your blood sugar more frequently and carry treatment supplies with you.

What causes high blood sugar?

High blood sugar (hyperglycemia) can result from illness, stress, overeating, insufficient insulin doses, or medication issues. Long-term high blood sugar levels can lead to serious health complications. Symptoms may include fatigue, thirst, blurred vision, increased urination, and difficulty managing blood sugar during illness.

How can I treat high blood sugar?

To lower high blood sugar, consider increasing physical activity, adjusting medication doses, adhering to your diabetes meal plan, and monitoring blood sugar levels closely. Consult your doctor for personalized advice on managing high blood sugar effectively.

How do carbs affect blood sugar?

Carbohydrates affect blood sugar levels more than proteins or fats. However, you can still include carbs in your diet while managing diabetes. Determine your carb goals based on factors like age, weight, activity level, and health status. Counting carbs and choosing appropriate portions can help regulate blood sugar levels effectively.

What is the A1C test?

The A1C test measures average blood sugar levels over the past 2-3 months. It complements regular blood sugar monitoring and provides insights into long-term glucose control. Aim for an A1C level between 7% and 8%, although targets may vary based on individual factors. Work with your doctor to establish personalized A1C goals.

What else can I do to help manage my blood sugar levels?

In addition to regular blood sugar monitoring and medication adherence, focus on maintaining a healthy diet, engaging in regular physical activity, and staying hydrated.

Track your food intake, practice portion control, and prioritize low-calorie, nutrient-dense foods. Avoid skipping meals, limit alcohol consumption, and seek support from healthcare professionals for personalized guidance on blood sugar management.

Importance of Diet in Diabetes Management

Diet plays a crucial role in diabetes management, impacting blood sugar levels, weight management, and overall health. Here's why dietary choices are essential for individuals with diabetes:

Blood Sugar Control: The foods you eat directly affect your blood sugar levels. Carbohydrates, in particular, have the most significant impact on blood sugar because they are broken down into glucose during digestion. By monitoring carbohydrate intake and choosing low-glycemic index foods, individuals with diabetes can better manage blood sugar levels and minimize spikes.

Weight Management: Maintaining a healthy weight is important for managing diabetes, as excess body weight can contribute to insulin resistance and complications.

A balanced diet that includes plenty of fruits, vegetables, lean proteins, and whole grains can help control calorie intake and support weight loss or weight maintenance efforts.

Heart Health: Diabetes increases the risk of cardiovascular disease, so it's essential to follow a heart-healthy diet. This includes reducing intake of saturated and trans fats, cholesterol, and sodium, while prioritizing unsaturated fats, fiber-rich foods, and omega-3 fatty acids. These dietary choices can help lower cholesterol levels, reduce blood pressure, and protect against heart disease.

Glycemic Control: Consistently choosing foods with a low glycemic index can help stabilize blood sugar levels and prevent sudden spikes and crashes. Foods with a low glycemic index, such as whole grains, legumes, and non-starchy vegetables, are digested more slowly, resulting in a gradual rise in blood sugar levels.

Nutrient Intake: Diabetes can increase the risk of nutrient deficiencies, so it's important to focus on nutrient-dense foods that provide essential vitamins, minerals, and antioxidants. A well-balanced diet that includes a variety of fruits, vegetables, whole grains, lean proteins, and healthy fats can help meet nutritional needs and support overall health.

Meal Timing and Portion Control: Consistency in meal timing and portion control is essential for managing blood sugar levels and preventing overeating. Eating regular, balanced meals and snacks throughout the day can help regulate appetite, prevent blood sugar fluctuations, and maintain energy levels.

Blood Pressure Management: High blood pressure is common in individuals with diabetes and can increase the risk of complications. Following a diet rich in fruits, vegetables, whole grains, and low-fat dairy products while limiting sodium intake can help lower blood pressure and reduce the risk of cardiovascular disease.

Individualized Approach: There is no one-size-fits-all diet for diabetes management. Each person's dietary needs and preferences are unique, so it's essential to work with a registered dietitian or healthcare provider to develop a personalized eating plan that meets individual goals and lifestyle factors.

How Age Impacts Diabetes Management

As we age, managing diabetes becomes increasingly important for maintaining overall health and well-being. Age can influence various aspects of diabetes management, including treatment strategies, lifestyle changes, and risk factors for complications. Here's how age impacts diabetes management:

Changes in Metabolism: With age, metabolism naturally slows down, making it more challenging to maintain stable blood sugar levels. This can necessitate adjustments to medication doses, dietary habits, and physical activity levels to accommodate changes in insulin sensitivity and glucose metabolism.

Comorbidities and Complications: As individuals age, they are more likely to develop other health conditions, such as hypertension, cardiovascular disease, and kidney disease, which can complicate diabetes management. Managing diabetes becomes part of a broader approach to overall health, requiring coordinated care and monitoring for comorbidities and complications.

Medication Management: Older adults may be taking multiple medications for various health conditions, increasing the risk of medication interactions and adverse effects. Healthcare providers must carefully consider the choice and dosing of diabetes medications to minimize risks while effectively managing blood sugar levels.

Nutritional Needs: Nutritional needs may change with age, affecting dietary choices and meal planning for individuals with diabetes. Older adults may require adjustments to their diet to accommodate changes in appetite, digestion, and nutrient absorption, while still supporting blood sugar control and overall health.

Physical Activity Levels: Aging can lead to changes in physical function and mobility, impacting the ability to engage in regular exercise and physical activity.

Finding enjoyable and accessible forms of exercise becomes essential for managing blood sugar levels, promoting cardiovascular health, and maintaining muscle strength and flexibility.

Cognitive Function: Cognitive function may decline with age, affecting the ability to adhere to diabetes management tasks, such as medication adherence, blood sugar monitoring, and meal planning. Caregiver support, simplified treatment regimens, and assistive technologies can help older adults manage diabetes effectively despite cognitive challenges.

Social Support and Lifestyle Factors: Social support networks and lifestyle factors, such as living arrangements, access to healthcare services, and financial resources, can significantly influence diabetes management outcomes in older adults. Engaging with support groups, community resources, and healthcare professionals can provide valuable support and guidance for managing diabetes effectively.

Individualized Care: Diabetes management in older adults requires a personalized approach that considers individual health status, preferences, and goals. Healthcare providers should collaborate with older adults and their caregivers to develop tailored treatment plans that prioritize quality of life, functional independence, and overall well-being.

Tips for Managing Diabetes in Your 50s and Beyond

Entering your 50s brings new considerations for managing diabetes effectively. As your body undergoes changes with age, it's essential to adapt your diabetes management strategies to maintain optimal health and well-being. Here are some practical tips for managing diabetes in your 50s and beyond:

Regular Health Check-ups: Schedule regular check-ups with your healthcare provider to monitor your blood sugar levels, blood pressure, cholesterol levels, kidney function, and other key health indicators.

Stay Active: Regular physical activity is crucial for managing diabetes and promoting overall health. Aim for at least 150 minutes of moderate-intensity aerobic activity per week, such as brisk walking, swimming, or cycling. Incorporate strength training exercises to maintain muscle mass and improve insulin sensitivity.

Healthy Eating Habits: Focus on a balanced diet rich in fruits, vegetables, whole grains, lean proteins, and healthy fats. Be mindful of portion sizes and carbohydrate intake to help regulate blood sugar levels. Consider working with a registered dietitian to develop a personalized meal plan that meets your nutritional needs and diabetes management goals.

Medication Adherence: Take your diabetes medications as prescribed by your healthcare provider. It's essential to adhere to your medication regimen to maintain stable blood sugar levels and prevent complications. If you have any concerns or experience side effects, discuss them with your healthcare provider promptly.

Monitor Blood Sugar Levels: Regularly monitor your blood sugar levels at home using a glucometer or continuous glucose monitor (CGM). Keep track of your readings and share them with your healthcare provider during check-ups. Monitoring blood sugar levels allows for adjustments to your treatment plan as needed to maintain optimal control.

Manage Stress: Chronic stress can affect blood sugar levels and overall health. Practice stress-reduction techniques such as deep breathing, meditation, yoga, or engaging in hobbies and activities you enjoy. Prioritize self-care and make time for relaxation to support your emotional well-being.

Quit Smoking: If you smoke, quitting is one of the best things you can do for your health, especially when managing diabetes. Smoking can worsen insulin resistance, increase the risk of cardiovascular complications, and impair circulation. Seek support from healthcare professionals or smoking cessation programs to quit successfully.

Get Enough Sleep: Aim for seven to nine hours of quality sleep per night. Poor sleep habits can disrupt hormone levels, including insulin, and affect blood sugar control. Establish a bedtime routine, create a comfortable sleep environment, and limit caffeine and electronic device use before bed to improve sleep quality.

Stay Informed: Stay up-to-date on diabetes management guidelines, new treatment options, and lifestyle recommendations. Educate yourself about diabetes and its complications, and ask questions during healthcare appointments to ensure you have a clear understanding of your condition and treatment plan.

Build a Support Network: Surround yourself with a supportive network of family, friends, and healthcare professionals who can provide encouragement, guidance, and assistance as needed. Joining diabetes support groups or online communities can also connect you with others who understand your experiences and challenges.

what food to eat and avoid

When managing diabetes, making wise food choices is essential for controlling blood sugar levels and promoting overall health. Here are some general guidelines on foods to eat and foods to avoid for individuals with diabetes:

Foods to Eat:

Non-Starchy Vegetables: Include a variety of non-starchy vegetables such as leafy greens, broccoli, cauliflower, peppers, and tomatoes in your meals. These vegetables are low in carbohydrates and calories but rich in fiber, vitamins, and minerals.

Whole Grains: Choose whole grains over refined grains to increase fiber intake and improve blood sugar control. Examples include brown rice, quinoa, barley, oats, and whole wheat bread or pasta.

Lean Proteins: Opt for lean sources of protein such as skinless poultry, fish, tofu, legumes, eggs, and low-fat dairy products. Protein-rich foods can help stabilize blood sugar levels and promote satiety.

Healthy Fats: Incorporate healthy fats into your diet, such as olive oil, avocado, nuts, seeds, and fatty fish like salmon and mackerel. These fats provide essential nutrients and help improve heart health.

Fruits: Enjoy fruits in moderation, focusing on lower glycemic options such as berries, apples, oranges, and cherries. Limit portions and pair fruits with protein or fiber to minimize blood sugar spikes.

Beans and Legumes: Beans and legumes are excellent sources of protein, fiber, and complex carbohydrates. Include options like lentils, chickpeas, black beans, and kidney beans in soups, salads, and main dishes.

Dairy: Choose low-fat or fat-free dairy products such as milk, yogurt, and cheese to reduce saturated fat intake while still obtaining calcium and protein. Greek yogurt is a particularly good choice due to its high protein content and lower carbohydrate content.

Healthy Beverages: Stay hydrated with water, herbal tea, and sparkling water. Limit sugary beverages such as soda, fruit juice, and sweetened coffee drinks, as they can cause blood sugar spikes.

Foods to Avoid or Limit:

Refined Carbohydrates: Minimize consumption of foods made with refined grains and added sugars, including white bread, white rice, sugary cereals, pastries, and sweetened snacks. These foods can cause rapid increases in blood sugar levels.

Sugary Drinks: Avoid sugary beverages such as soda, fruit punch, energy drinks, and sweetened teas, as they can contribute to weight gain and worsen blood sugar control.

Processed Foods: Reduce intake of processed and convenience foods high in unhealthy fats, sodium, and added sugars. Examples include fried foods, fast food, packaged snacks, and frozen meals.

Saturated and Trans Fats: Limit consumption of foods high in saturated and trans fats, such as fatty cuts of meat, processed meats, full-fat dairy products, and fried foods. These fats can increase the risk of heart disease and insulin resistance.

High-Sodium Foods: Cut back on high-sodium foods like canned soups, salty snacks, processed meats, and fast food, as excessive sodium intake can raise blood pressure and increase the risk of heart disease.

Sweetened Condiments: Avoid or use sparingly condiments and sauces high in added sugars, such as ketchup, barbecue sauce, and sweetened salad dressings. Choose low-sugar or homemade alternatives whenever possible.

Alcohol: Limit alcohol consumption and be mindful of its effects on blood sugar levels. Choose light beer, dry wine, or spirits mixed with calorie-free mixers, and drink in moderation.

CHAPTER 2:
Breakfast Recipes

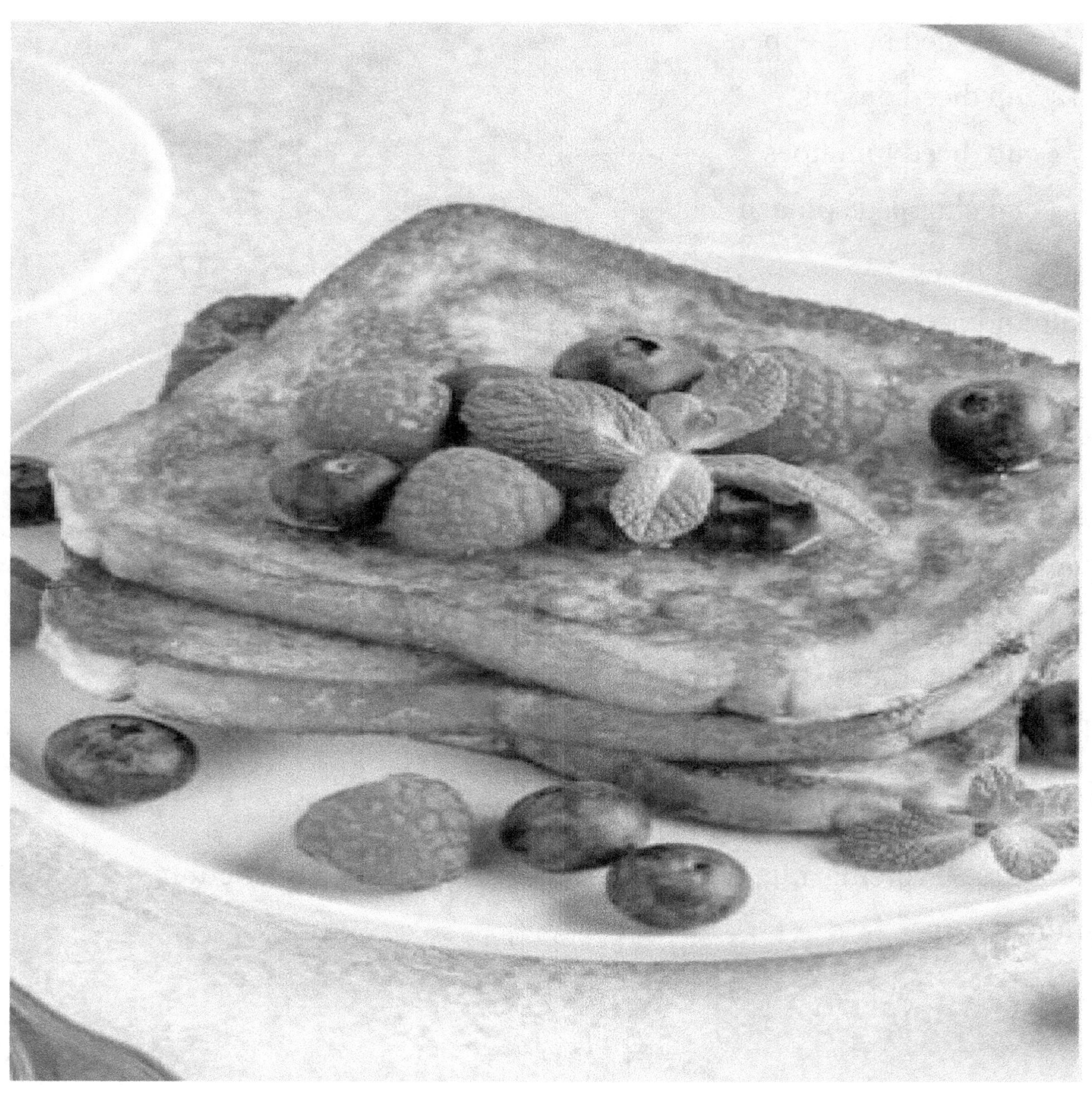

Veggie Omelette

Prep Time: 10 minutes: Cooking Time: 10 minutes: Serving Size: 1

Ingredients:

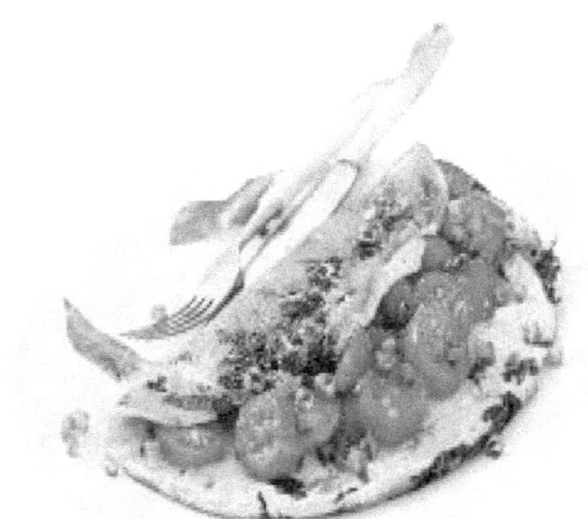

- 2 large eggs
- 1/4 cup diced bell peppers
- 1/4 cup diced onions
- 1/4 cup diced tomatoes
- 1/4 cup chopped spinach
- 1 tsp olive oil
- Salt and pepper to taste

Instructions:

1. Heat olive oil in a non-stick skillet over medium heat.
2. In a bowl, whisk eggs and season with salt and pepper.
3. Pour eggs into the skillet and let them cook for 2 minutes.
4. Sprinkle veggies evenly over the eggs.
5. Cook for another 2-3 minutes until the omelette is set.
6. Fold the omelette in half and serve.

Nutritional Information (per serving):

Calories: 200, Protein: 14g, Carbohydrates: 10g, Fiber: 3g, Sodium: 150mg, Potassium: 320mg

Greek Yogurt Parfait

Prep Time: 5 minutes: Serving Size: 1

Ingredients:

- 1/2 cup plain Greek yogurt
- 1/4 cup mixed berries (strawberries, blueberries, raspberries)
- 1 tbsp chopped nuts (almonds, walnuts)
- 1 tsp honey (optional)

Instructions:

1. In a glass or bowl, layer Greek yogurt, mixed berries, and chopped nuts.
2. Drizzle honey on top if desired.
3. Serve immediately.

Nutritional Information (per serving):

Calories: 180, Protein: 18g, Carbohydrates: 18g, Fiber: 4g, Sugar: 12g, Sodium: 50mg, Potassium: 250mg

Avocado Toast

Prep Time: 5 minutes: Cooking Time: 5 minutes: Serving Size: 1

Ingredients:

- 1 slice whole grain bread
- 1/2 ripe avocado
- 1 tsp lemon juice
- Salt and pepper to taste

Instructions:

1. Toast the bread until golden brown.
2. In a bowl, mash the avocado with lemon juice, salt, and pepper.

3. Spread the mashed avocado onto the toasted bread.

4. Serve immediately.

Nutritional Information (per serving):

Calories: 220, Protein: 5g, Carbohydrates: 20g, Fiber: 7g, Sugar: 1g, Sodium: 150mg, Potassium: 350mg

Berry Smoothie

Prep Time: 5 minutes: Serving Size: 1

Ingredients:

- 1/2 cup mixed berries (strawberries, blueberries, raspberries)
- 1/2 cup unsweetened almond milk
- 1/4 cup plain Greek yogurt
- 1 tbsp chia seeds
- 1 tsp honey (optional)

Instructions:

1. In a blender, combine mixed berries, almond milk, Greek yogurt, and chia seeds.

2. Blend until smooth.

3. Sweeten with honey if desired.

4. Serve immediately.

Nutritional Information (per serving): Calories: 180, Protein: 10g, Carbohydrates: 20g, Fiber: 7g, Sugar: 10g, Sodium: 100mg, Potassium: 300mg

Quinoa Breakfast Bowl

Prep Time: 10 minutes: Cooking Time: 15 minutes: Serving Size: 1

Ingredients

- 1/4 cup quinoa
- 1/2 cup water
- 1/4 cup diced mango
- 1/4 cup diced strawberries
- 1 tbsp chopped almonds
- 1 tsp honey (optional)

Instructions:

1. Rinse quinoa under cold water.
2. In a saucepan, bring water to a boil and add quinoa.
3. Reduce heat, cover, and simmer for 12-15 minutes until quinoa is cooked and water is absorbed.
4. Fluff quinoa with a fork and transfer to a bowl.
5. Top with diced mango, strawberries, and chopped almonds.
6. Drizzle honey on top if desired.

Nutritional Information (per serving):

Calories: 280, Protein: 8g, Carbohydrates: 45g, Fiber: 6g, Sugar: 15g, Sodium: 10mg, Potassium: 350mg

Chia Seed Pudding

Prep Time: 5 minutes: Chilling Time: 4 hours: Serving Size: 1

Ingredients:

- 2 tbsp chia seeds
- 1/2 cup unsweetened almond milk
- 1/4 tsp vanilla extract
- 1 tsp honey (optional)

Instructions:

1. In a bowl, mix chia seeds, almond milk, vanilla extract, and honey.
2. Cover and refrigerate for at least 4 hours or overnight until thickened.
3. Stir well before serving.
4. Top with berries or nuts if desired.

Nutritional Information (per serving): Calories: 150, Protein: 5g, Carbohydrates: 12g, Fiber: 8g, Sugar: 3g, Sodium: 70mg, Potassium: 100mg}

Smoked Salmon Breakfast Wrap

Prep Time: 10 minutes: Cooking Time: 5 minutes: Serving Size: 1

Ingredients:

- 1 whole grain tortilla
- 2 oz smoked salmon
- 1/4 avocado, sliced
- 1/4 cup baby spinach leaves
- 1 tbsp Greek yogurt

Instructions:

1. Place tortilla on a flat surface.
2. Layer smoked salmon, avocado slices, spinach leaves, and Greek yogurt on the tortilla.
3. Roll up the tortilla tightly.
4. Slice in half and serve.

Nutritional Information (per serving):

Calories: 280, Protein: 15g, Carbohydrates: 20g, Fiber: 6g, Sugar: 1g, Sodium: 450mg, Potassium: 450mg

Banana Nut Overnight Oats

Prep Time: 5 minutes: Chilling Time: 4 hours: Serving Size: 1

Ingredients:

- 1/2 cup rolled oats
- 1/2 cup unsweetened almond milk
- 1/2 ripe banana, mashed
- 1 tbsp chopped walnuts
- 1 tsp honey (optional)

Instructions:

1. In a jar or bowl, mix rolled oats, almond milk, mashed banana, chopped walnuts, and honey.
2. Cover and refrigerate for at least 4 hours or overnight.
3. Before serving, stir well and add more almond milk if desired.
4. Enjoy cold.

Nutritional Information (per serving): Calories: 300, Protein: 8g, Carbohydrates: 40g, Fiber: 7g, Sugar: 10g, Sodium: 80mg, Potassium: 350mg}

Peanut Butter Banana Smoothie

Prep Time: 5 minutes: Serving Size: 1

Ingredients:

- 1 ripe banana
- 1 tbsp natural peanut butter
- 1/2 cup unsweetened almond milk
- 1/4 cup plain Greek yogurt
- 1 tsp honey (optional)

Instructions:

1. In a blender, combine banana, peanut butter, almond milk, Greek yogurt, and honey.
2. Blend until smooth.
3. Pour into a glass and serve immediately.

Nutritional Information (per serving):

Calories: 280, Protein: 12g, Carbohydrates: 30g, Fiber: 5g, Sugar: 15g, Sodium: 180mg, Potassium: 450mg.

Cottage Cheese Pancakes

Prep Time: 10 minutes: Cooking Time: 10 minutes: Serving Size: 2 pancakes

Ingredients:

- 1/2 cup low-fat cottage cheese
- 2 large eggs
- 1/4 cup almond flour
- 1/2 tsp baking powder
- 1/2 tsp vanilla extract

Instructions:

1. In a blender, combine cottage cheese, eggs, almond flour, baking powder, and vanilla extract.
2. Blend until smooth.
3. Heat a non-stick skillet over medium heat and lightly grease with cooking spray.
4. Pour 1/4 cup of batter onto the skillet for each pancake.
5. Cook for 2-3 minutes until bubbles form on the surface, then flip and cook for another 1-2 minutes until golden brown.
6. Repeat with the remaining batter.
7. Serve warm with fresh berries or a drizzle of sugar-free syrup.

Nutritional Information (per serving, 2 pancakes):

Calories: 250, Protein: 22g, Carbohydrates: 10g, Fiber: 2g, Sugar: 3gSodium: , 400mg, Potassium: 300mg}

Tofu Scramble

Prep Time: 10 minutes: Cooking Time: 10 minutes: Serving Size: 1

Ingredients:

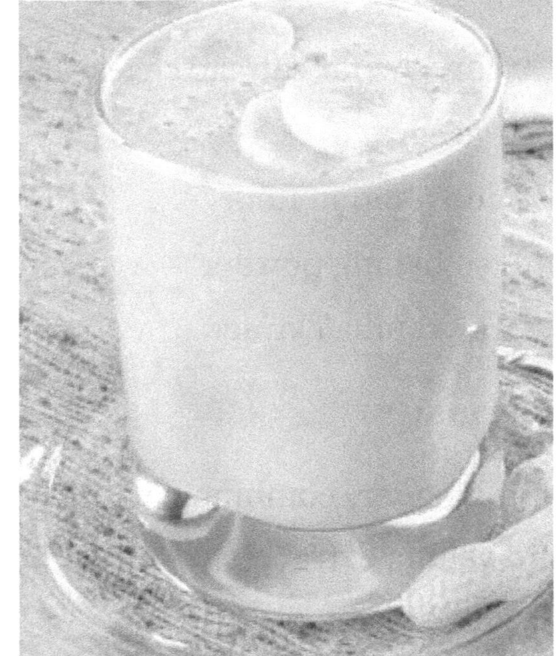

- 100g firm tofu, crumbled
- 1/4 cup diced bell peppers
- 1/4 cup diced onions
- 1/4 cup diced tomatoes
- 1/4 tsp turmeric
- 1/4 tsp garlic powder
- Salt and pepper to taste
- 1 tsp olive oil

Instructions:

1. Heat olive oil in a skillet over medium heat.
2. Add bell peppers, onions, and tomatoes, and cook until softened.
3. Add crumbled tofu to the skillet and sprinkle with turmeric, garlic powder, salt, and pepper.
4. Cook for 5-7 minutes, stirring occasionally, until tofu is heated through and slightly golden.
5. Serve hot with whole grain toast or tortilla.

Nutritional Information (per serving):

Calories: 210, Protein: 15g, Carbohydrates: 10g, Fiber: 3g, Sugar: 4g, Sodium: 150mg, Potassium: 400mg

Apple Cinnamon Oatmeal

Prep Time: 5 minutes: Cooking Time: 10 minutes: Serving Size: 1

Ingredients:

- 1/2 cup rolled oats
- 1 cup water
- 1/2 apple, diced
- 1/2 tsp cinnamon
- 1 tbsp chopped walnuts

Instructions:

1. In a saucepan, bring water to a boil.
2. Stir in rolled oats, diced apple, and cinnamon.
3. Reduce heat to low and simmer for 5-7 minutes, stirring occasionally, until oats are creamy and tender.
4. Remove from heat and let stand for 2 minutes.
5. Transfer to a bowl and sprinkle with chopped walnuts.
6. Serve hot.

Nutritional Information (per serving):

Calories: 240, Protein: 7g: 35g, Fiber: 6g, Sugar: 10g, Sodium: 5mg, Potassium: 220mg}

Kale and Mushroom Frittata

Prep Time: 10 minutes: Cooking Time: 20 minutes: Serving Size: 1

Ingredients:

- 2 large eggs
- 1/2 cup chopped kale
- 1/4 cup sliced mushrooms
- 1/4 cup diced onions
- 1/4 cup shredded low-fat mozzarella cheese
- 1 tsp olive oil
- Salt and pepper to taste

Instructions:

1. Preheat the oven to 350°F (175°C).
2. In a bowl, whisk eggs and season with salt and pepper.
3. Heat olive oil in an oven-safe skillet over medium heat.
4. Add onions and mushrooms, and cook until softened.
5. Add chopped kale to the skillet and cook until wilted.
6. Pour eggs into the skillet and sprinkle mozzarella cheese on top.
7. Transfer the skillet to the oven and bake for 15 minutes or until the frittata is set.
8. Slice and serve.

Nutritional Information (per serving):

Calories: 280, Protein: 18g, Carbohydrates: 10g, Fiber: 3g, Sugar: 4g, Sodium: 350mg, Potassium: 450mg}

Whole Wheat Pancakes

Prep Time: 10 minutes: Cooking Time: 10 minutes: Serving Size: 2 pancakes

Ingredients:

- 1/2 cup whole wheat flour
- 1/2 cup unsweetened almond milk
- 1 large egg
- 1 tbsp unsweetened applesauce
- 1 tsp baking powder
- 1/2 tsp vanilla extract

Instructions:

1. In a bowl, whisk together whole wheat flour, almond milk, egg, applesauce, baking powder, and vanilla extract until smooth.
2. Heat a non-stick skillet or griddle over medium heat and lightly grease with cooking spray.
3. Pour 1/4 cup of batter onto the skillet for each pancake.
4. Cook for 2-3 minutes until bubbles form on the surface, then flip and cook for another 1-2 minutes until golden brown.
5. Repeat with the remaining batter.
6. Serve warm with sugar-free syrup or fresh fruit.

Nutritional Information (per serving, 2 pancakes):

Calories: 220, Protein: 9g, Carbohydrates: 30g, Fiber: 5g, Sugar: 1g, Sodium: 300mg, Potassium: 200mg}

Tuna Salad Stuffed Avocado

Prep Time: 10 minutes: Serving Size: 1

Ingredients:

- 1 ripe avocado
- 1/2 cup canned tuna, drained
- 1 tbsp plain Greek yogurt
- 1/4 cup diced cucumber
- 1/4 cup diced tomatoes
- 1 tbsp chopped cilantro
- 1 tsp lemon juice
- Salt and pepper to taste

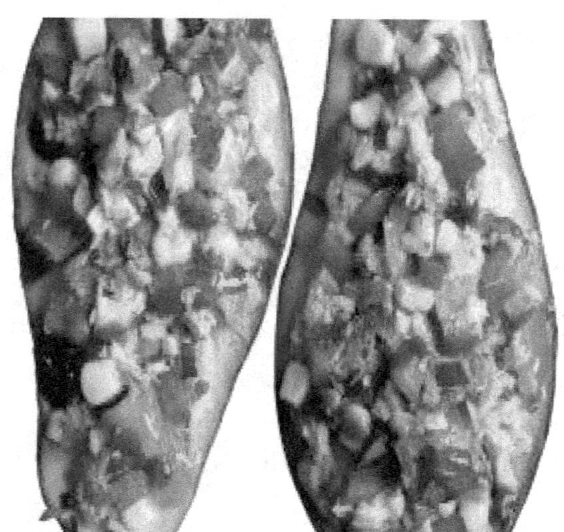

Instructions:

1. Cut the avocado in half and remove the pit.
2. In a bowl, mix tuna, Greek yogurt, cucumber, tomatoes, cilantro, lemon juice, salt, and pepper.
3. Scoop the tuna salad into the avocado halves.
4. Serve immediately.

Nutritional Information (per serving):

Calories: 320, Protein: 20g, Carbohydrates: 15g, Fiber: 9g, Sugar: 2g, Sodium: 300mg, Potassium: 700mg}

Berry Chia Seed Smoothie Bowl

Prep Time: 5 minutes, Serving Size: 1

Ingredients:

- 1/2 cup mixed berries (strawberries, blueberries, raspberries)
- 1/2 cup unsweetened almond milk
- 2 tbsp chia seeds
- 1 tbsp almond butter
- 1 tsp honey (optional)

Instructions:

1. In a blender, combine mixed berries, almond milk, chia seeds, almond butter, and honey.
2. Blend until smooth.
3. Pour into a bowl and top with additional berries or nuts if desired.
4. Serve immediately.

Nutritional Information (per serving):

Calories: 290, Protein: 10g, Carbohydrates: 20g, Fiber: 10g, Sugar: 8g, Sodium: 100mg, Potassium: 300mg

Egg White Breakfast Burrito

Prep Time: 10 minutes: Cooking Time: 10 minutes: Serving Size: 1

Ingredients:

- 2 large egg whites
- 1 whole grain tortilla
- 1/4 cup black beans, drained and rinsed
- 1/4 avocado, sliced

- 1/4 cup salsa

Instructions:

1. In a non-stick skillet, cook egg whites over medium heat until set.
2. Warm the tortilla in the skillet or microwave.
3. Layer cooked egg whites, black beans, avocado slices, and salsa on the tortilla.
4. Roll up the tortilla tightly.
5. Slice in half and serve.

Nutritional Information (per serving): Calories: 280, Protein: 15g, Carbohydrates: 30g, Fiber: 10g, Sugar: 2g, Sodium: 350mg, Potassium: 450mg}

Sweet Potato Breakfast Hash

Prep Time: 10 minutes: Cooking Time: 20 minutes: Serving Size: 1

Ingredients:

- 1 small sweet potato, peeled and diced
- 1/4 cup diced bell peppers
- 1/4 cup diced onions
- 1/4 cup black beans, drained and rinsed
- 1/4 avocado, sliced
- 1 tsp olive oil
- Salt and pepper to taste

Instructions:

1. Heat olive oil in a skillet over medium heat.
2. Add sweet potatoes, bell peppers, and onions to the skillet.
3. Cook until sweet potatoes are tender and lightly browned, about 15 minutes.
4. Stir in black beans and cook for an additional 3-5 minutes.

5. Season with salt and pepper.
6. Serve hot, topped with sliced avocado.

Nutritional Information (per serving):

Calories: 320, Protein: 8g, Carbohydrates: 45g, Fiber: 12g, Sugar: 8g, Sodium: 200mg, Potassium: 700mg}

Nutty Banana Porridge

Prep Time: 5 minutes: Cooking Time: 10 minutes: Serving Size: 1

Ingredients:

- 1/2 cup rolled oats
- 1 cup unsweetened almond milk
- 1/2 ripe banana, mashed
- 1 tbsp chopped walnuts
- 1 tsp ground cinnamon

Instructions:

1. In a saucepan, bring almond milk to a gentle boil.
2. Stir in rolled oats and reduce heat to low.
3. Cook for 5-7 minutes, stirring occasionally, until oats are creamy and tender.
4. Stir in mashed banana, chopped walnuts, and ground cinnamon.
5. Cook for another 2-3 minutes until heated through.
6. Transfer to a bowl and serve hot.

Nutritional Information (per serving):

Calories: 290, Protein: 9g, Carbohydrates: 40g, Fiber: 7g, Sugar: 8g, Sodium: 110mg, Potassium: 370mg

Quinoa Breakfast Porridge

Prep Time: 5 minutes: Cooking Time: 15 minutes: Serving Size: 1

Ingredients:

- 1/4 cup quinoa, rinsed
- 1/2 cup unsweetened almond milk
- 1/2 cup water
- 1/2 apple, diced
- 1 tbsp raisins
- 1/4 tsp ground cinnamon

Instructions:

1. In a saucepan, combine quinoa, almond milk, water, diced apple, raisins, and ground cinnamon.
2. Bring to a boil, then reduce heat to low and simmer for 12-15 minutes until quinoa is cooked and liquid is absorbed.
3. Stir occasionally to prevent sticking.
4. Remove from heat and let stand for 2 minutes.
5. Transfer to a bowl and serve warm.

Nutritional Information (per serving):

Calories: 270, Protein: 8g, Carbohydrates: 50g, Fiber: 6g, Sugar: 18g, Sodium: 90mg, Potassium: 380mg}

High-Fiber Cereal Bowl

Prep Time: 5 minutes: Serving Size: 1

Ingredients:

- 1/2 cup high-fiber cereal (check for sugar content)
- 1/2 cup unsweetened almond milk
- 1/4 cup mixed berries (strawberries, blueberries, raspberries)
- 1 tbsp chopped nuts (almonds, walnuts)

Instructions:

1. In a bowl, combine high-fiber cereal and unsweetened almond milk.

2. Top with mixed berries and chopped nuts.

3. Serve immediately.

Nutritional Information (per serving): Calories: 220, Protein: 6gCarbohydrates: 30g, Fiber: 10g, Sugar: 5g, Sodium: 120mg, Potassium: 250mg

Coconut Almond Millet Porridge

Prep Time: 5 minutes: Cooking Time: 20 minutes: Serving Size: 1

Ingredients:

- 1/4 cup millet
- 1 cup unsweetened coconut milk
- 1/2 cup water
- 1 tbsp unsweetened shredded coconut
- 1 tbsp chopped almonds
- 1/4 tsp vanilla extract
- 1 tsp maple syrup (optional)

Instructions:

1. Rinse the millet under cold water.

2. In a saucepan, combine millet, coconut milk, water, shredded coconut, chopped almonds, vanilla extract, and maple syrup (if using).

3. Bring the mixture to a boil, then reduce the heat to low.

4. Simmer uncovered for 15-20 minutes, stirring occasionally, until the millet is tender and the mixture thickens.

5. Remove from heat and let it sit for a few minutes to thicken further.

6. Transfer the porridge to a bowl and serve warm.

Nutritional Information (per serving): Calories: 320, Protein: 7g, Carbohydrates: 30g, Fiber: 5g, Sugar: 1g, Fat: 22g, Saturated Fat: 15g, Sodium: 20mg, Potassium: 210mg

Breakfast Tostada

Prep Time: 10 minutes: Cooking Time: 10 minutes: Serving Size: 1 tostada

Ingredients:

- 1 corn tortilla
- 1/4 cup black beans, drained and rinsed
- 1/4 avocado, sliced
- 1 egg
- 2 tbsp salsa
- Salt and pepper to taste
- Optional toppings: chopped cilantro, sliced jalapenos, crumbled feta cheese

Instructions:

1. Heat a non-stick skillet over medium heat.
2. Place the corn tortilla in the skillet and cook until lightly crisp on both sides, about 2-3 minutes per side.
3. In the meantime, heat the black beans in a small saucepan or microwave until warm.
4. Once the tortilla is crisp, remove it from the skillet and place it on a plate.
5. Spread warmed black beans over the tortilla.
6. In the same skillet, fry the egg to your desired doneness (such as sunny-side-up or scrambled).
7. Carefully place the cooked egg on top of the black beans.
8. Arrange sliced avocado on top of the egg.
9. Spoon salsa over the avocado.
10. Season with salt and pepper to taste.
11. If desired, garnish with chopped cilantro, sliced jalapenos, or crumbled feta cheese.
12. Serve immediately, with optional hot sauce on the side.

CHAPTER 3
Dinner Delights

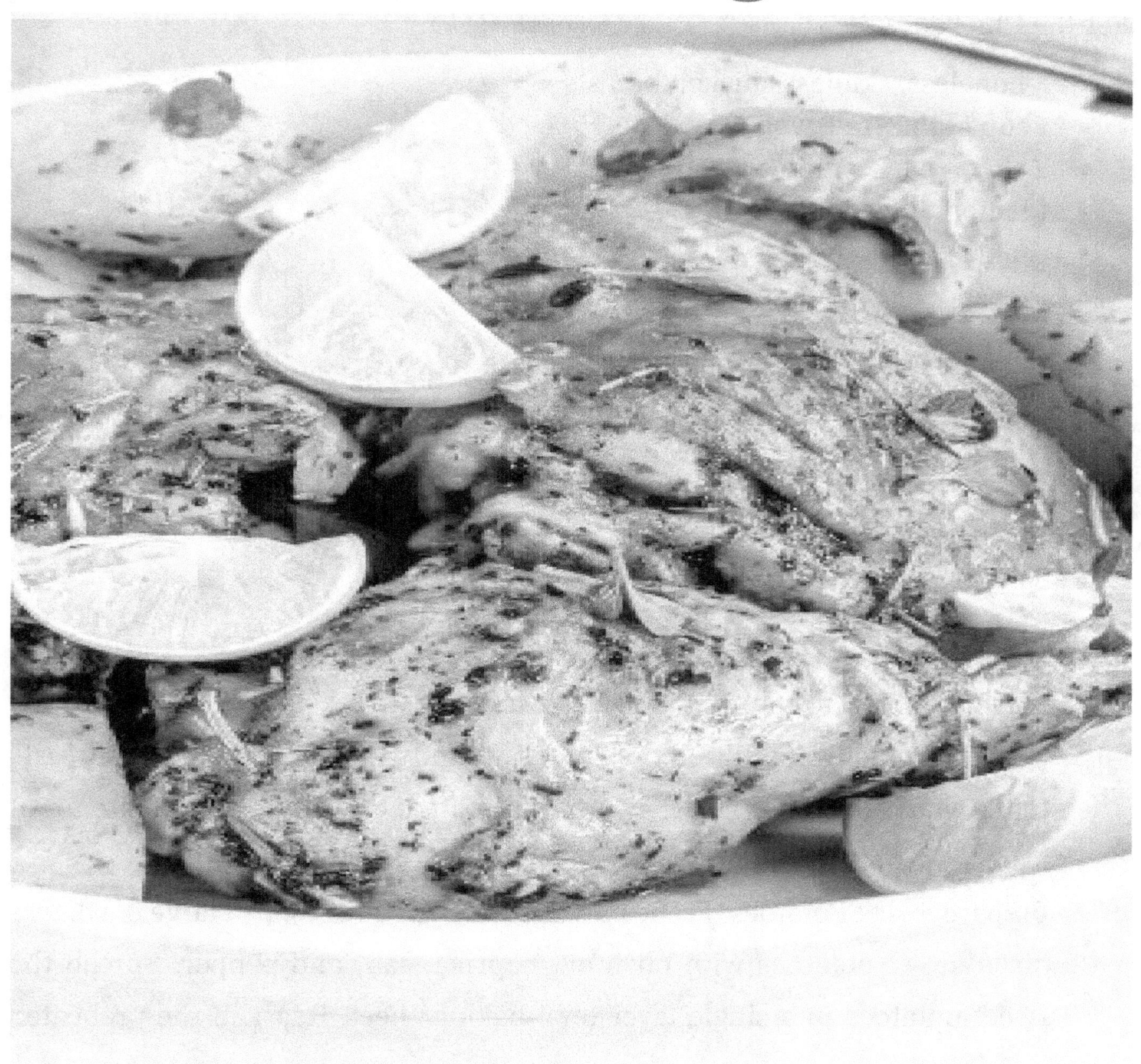

Grilled Chicken with Greek Yogurt Marinade and Roasted Sweet Potato

Prep Time: 15 minutes: Cooking Time: 25 minutes: Serving Size: 4

Ingredients:

For the Chicken:

- 4 boneless, skinless chicken breasts
- 1 cup plain Greek yogurt
- 2 cloves garlic, minced
- 1 lemon, juiced
- 1 tablespoon olive oil
- 1 teaspoon dried oregano
- Salt and pepper to taste

For the Sweet Potatoes:

- 2 large sweet potatoes, peeled and diced
- 1 tablespoon olive oil
- 1 teaspoon paprika
- Salt and pepper to taste

Method of Preparation:

1. Marinate the Chicken: In a bowl, mix together Greek yogurt, minced garlic, lemon juice, olive oil, dried oregano, salt, and pepper. Add chicken breasts to the marinade, ensuring they are well coated. Cover and refrigerate for at least 1 hour or overnight.

2. Prepare Sweet Potatoes: Preheat oven to 400°F (200°C). In a large bowl, toss diced sweet potatoes with olive oil, paprika, salt, and pepper. Spread the sweet potatoes in a single layer on a baking sheet. Roast in the preheated

oven for 20-25 minutes or until tender and lightly browned, flipping halfway through cooking.

3. Grill the Chicken: Preheat grill to medium-high heat. Remove chicken breasts from the marinade, shaking off any excess. Grill the chicken for 6-7 minutes per side or until cooked through and no longer pink in the center.

4. Serve: Serve the grilled chicken with roasted sweet potatoes on the side.

Nutritional Value (per serving): Calories: 350, Total Fat: 10g, Saturated Fat: 2g, Cholesterol: 90mg, Sodium: 200mg, Total Carbohydrates: 25g, Dietary Fiber: 4g, Sugars: 7g, Protein: 35g

Salmon with Lemon Dill Sauce and Asparagus

Prep Time: 10 minutes: Cooking Time: 15 minutes: Serving Size: 4

Ingredients:

For the Salmon:

- 4 salmon fillets (about 6 ounces each), skin-on or skinless
- 2 tablespoons olive oil
- Salt and pepper to taste

For the Lemon Dill Sauce:

- 1/4 cup plain Greek yogurt
- 2 tablespoons fresh dill, chopped
- 1 tablespoon lemon juice
- 1 teaspoon lemon zest
- Salt and pepper to taste

For the Asparagus:

- 1 bunch asparagus, woody ends trimmed
- 1 tablespoon olive oil
- Salt and pepper to taste

Method of Preparation:

1. Preheat Oven: Preheat the oven to 400°F (200°C).

2. Prepare Salmon: Pat the salmon fillets dry with paper towels. Rub them with olive oil and season with salt and pepper.

3. Roast Salmon and Asparagus: Place the seasoned salmon fillets and trimmed asparagus on a baking sheet lined with parchment paper. Drizzle olive oil over the asparagus and season with salt and pepper. Roast in the preheated oven for 12-15 minutes, or until the salmon is cooked through and the asparagus is tender.

4. Make Lemon Dill Sauce: In a small bowl, mix together Greek yogurt, chopped dill, lemon juice, lemon zest, salt, and pepper to make the sauce.

5. Serve: Serve the roasted salmon and asparagus hot, drizzled with the lemon dill sauce.

Nutritional Value (per serving): Calories: 320, Total Fat: 20g, Saturated Fat: 3g, Cholesterol: 80mg, Sodium: 150mg, Total Carbohydrates: 4g, Dietary Fiber: 2g, Sugars: 1g, Protein: 30g

Lentil Bolognese with Whole-Wheat Spaghetti

Prep Time: 10 minutes: Cooking Time: 30 minutes: Serving Size: 4

Ingredients:

- 8 oz whole-wheat spaghetti
- 1 cup dried brown lentils
- 1 tablespoon olive oil
- 1 onion, finely chopped
- 2 cloves garlic, minced
- 1 carrot, diced
- 1 stalk celery, diced
- 1 can (14 oz) crushed tomatoes
- 1 teaspoon dried oregano
- Salt and pepper to taste
- Fresh parsley, chopped (for garnish)

Method of Preparation:

1. Cook whole-wheat spaghetti according to package instructions. Drain and set aside.

2. In a large skillet, heat olive oil over medium heat. Add onion, garlic, carrot, and celery. Sauté until vegetables are softened, about 5 minutes.

3. Add dried lentils, crushed tomatoes, dried oregano, salt, and pepper. Stir to combine.

4. Cover and simmer for 20-25 minutes, or until lentils are tender and the sauce has thickened.

5. Serve lentil Bolognese over cooked whole-wheat spaghetti. Garnish with chopped parsley.

Nutritional Value (per serving): Calories: 380, Total Fat: 5g, Saturated Fat: 1g, Cholesterol: 0mg, Sodium: 250mg, Total Carbohydrates: 70g, Dietary Fiber: 14g, Sugars: 7g, Protein: 19g

Turkey Taco Bowls with Black Beans, Corn, and Guacamole

Prep Time: 15 minutes: Cooking Time: 20 minutes: Serving Size: 4

Ingredients:

- 1 lb ground turkey
- 1 tablespoon olive oil
- 1 onion, diced
- 1 bell pepper, diced
- 1 cup corn kernels (fresh or frozen)
- 1 can (15 oz) black beans, drained and rinsed
- 1 teaspoon chili powder
- 1/2 teaspoon ground cumin
- Salt and pepper to taste
- 2 cups cooked brown rice
- Guacamole, for serving
- Fresh cilantro, chopped (for garnish)

Method of Preparation:

1. In a large skillet, heat olive oil over medium heat. Add diced onion and bell pepper. Sauté until softened, about 5 minutes.
2. Add ground turkey to the skillet. Cook until browned and cooked through, breaking it up with a spoon as it cooks.
3. Stir in corn kernels, black beans, chili powder, ground cumin, salt, and pepper. Cook for another 5 minutes to heat through.
4. To assemble taco bowls, divide cooked brown rice among serving bowls. Top with turkey mixture, guacamole, and chopped cilantro.

Nutritional Value (per serving): Calories: 450, Total Fat: 15g, Saturated Fat: 3g, Cholesterol: 60mg, Sodium: 350mg, Total Carbohydrates: 55g, Dietary Fiber: 10g, Sugars: 4g, Protein: 28g

One-Pan Lemon Garlic Shrimp with Broccoli and Quinoa

Prep Time: 10 minutes: Cooking Time: 20 minutes: Serving Size: 4

Ingredients:

- 1 cup quinoa, rinsed
- 1 3/4 cups water or vegetable broth
- 1 lb large shrimp, peeled and deveined
- 2 tablespoons olive oil
- 4 cloves garlic, minced
- 1 lemon, juiced and zested
- 2 cups broccoli florets
- Salt and pepper to taste
- Fresh parsley, chopped (for garnish)

Method of Preparation:

1. In a saucepan, bring water or vegetable broth to a boil. Add rinsed quinoa, reduce heat to low, cover, and simmer for 15-20 minutes, or until quinoa is cooked and liquid is absorbed.

2. In a large skillet, heat olive oil over medium heat. Add minced garlic and cook until fragrant, about 1 minute.

3. Add shrimp to the skillet in a single layer. Cook for 2-3 minutes per side, or until shrimp turn pink and opaque.

4. Add broccoli florets to the skillet with the shrimp. Cook for an additional 3-4 minutes, or until broccoli is tender-crisp.

5. Stir in lemon juice and zest. Season with salt and pepper to taste.

6. Serve lemon garlic shrimp and broccoli over cooked quinoa. Garnish with chopped parsley.

Nutritional Value (per serving): Calories: 350, Total Fat: 10g, Saturated Fat: 1.5g, Cholesterol: 180mg, Sodium: 400mg, Total Carbohydrates: 35g, Dietary Fiber: 6g, Sugars: 2g, Protein: 30g

Chicken Souvlaki with Greek Salad and Whole-Wheat Pita Bread

Prep Time: 15 minutes (plus marinating time): Cooking Time: 15 minutes: Serving Size: 4

Ingredients:

For the Chicken Souvlaki:

- 1 lb boneless, skinless chicken breasts, cut into bite-sized pieces
- 1/4 cup olive oil
- 2 cloves garlic, minced
- 1 lemon, juiced and zested
- 1 teaspoon dried oregano
- Salt and pepper to taste
- Wooden skewers, soaked in water for 30 minutes

For the Greek Salad:

- 2 large tomatoes, diced
- 1 cucumber, diced
- 1/2 red onion, thinly sliced
- 1/4 cup Kalamata olives, pitted
- 2 tablespoons extra-virgin olive oil
- 1 tablespoon red wine vinegar
- 1 teaspoon dried oregano
- Salt and pepper to taste
- 4 whole-wheat pita breads, warmed

Method of Preparation:

1. In a bowl, whisk together olive oil, minced garlic, lemon juice, lemon zest, dried oregano, salt, and pepper to make the marinade for the chicken.
2. Add the chicken pieces to the marinade, ensuring they are well coated. Cover and refrigerate for at least 30 minutes, or up to 4 hours.

3. While the chicken is marinating, prepare the Greek salad. In a large bowl, combine diced tomatoes, diced cucumber, thinly sliced red onion, and pitted Kalamata olives.

4. In a small bowl, whisk together extra-virgin olive oil, red wine vinegar, dried oregano, salt, and pepper to make the salad dressing. Pour the dressing over the salad ingredients and toss gently to coat.

5. Preheat grill or grill pan over medium-high heat. Thread marinated chicken pieces onto soaked wooden skewers.

6. Grill the chicken skewers for 4-5 minutes per side, or until cooked through and lightly charred.

7. Warm whole-wheat pita bread in the oven or on the grill for a few minutes.

8. Serve the grilled chicken souvlaki with Greek salad and warm whole-wheat pita bread on the side.

Nutritional Value (per serving): Calories: 380, Total Fat: 15g, Saturated Fat: 2.5g, Cholesterol: 80mg, Sodium: 400mg, Total Carbohydrates: 35g,Dietary Fiber: 6g, Sugars: 4g, Protein: 30g

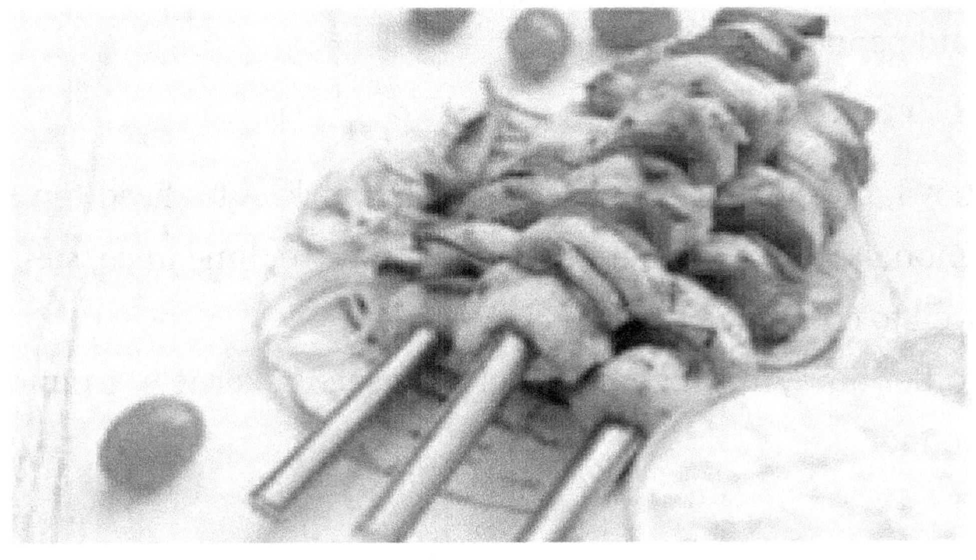

Black Bean and Corn Quesadillas with Avocado Salsa

Prep Time: 10 minutes: Cooking Time: 15 minutes: Serving Size: 4

Ingredients:

For the Quesadillas:

- 8 whole-wheat tortillas
- 1 can (15 oz) black beans, drained and rinsed
- 1 cup corn kernels (fresh or frozen)
- 1 cup shredded cheese (such as cheddar or Monterey Jack)
- 1 teaspoon ground cumin
- Salt and pepper to taste
- Cooking spray or olive oil for cooking

For the Avocado Salsa:

- 1 ripe avocado, diced
- 1 tomato, diced
- 1/4 cup red onion, finely chopped
- 1 jalapeño, seeded and finely chopped (optional)
- 2 tablespoons fresh cilantro, chopped
- 1 lime, juiced
- Salt and pepper to taste

Method of Preparation:

1. In a bowl, mash the diced avocado with a fork. Add diced tomato, chopped red onion, jalapeño (if using), chopped cilantro, lime juice, salt, and pepper. Mix well to combine. Set aside.

2. In another bowl, mix together black beans, corn kernels, ground cumin, salt, and pepper.

3. Heat a large skillet or griddle over medium heat. Place one tortilla in the skillet and spread a layer of the black bean and corn mixture on half of the tortilla. Sprinkle shredded cheese over the bean mixture and fold the tortilla in half.

4. Cook the quesadilla for 2-3 minutes on each side, or until the tortilla is crispy and golden brown, and the cheese is melted. Repeat with the remaining tortillas and filling ingredients.

5. Cut the cooked quesadillas into wedges and serve hot with the avocado salsa on the side.

Nutritional Value (per serving): Calories: 380, Total Fat: 15g, Saturated Fat: 5g, Cholesterol: 20mg, Sodium: 500mg, Total Carbohydrates: 50g, Dietary Fiber: 12g, Sugars: 3g, Protein: 15g

Tofu Teriyaki with Brown Rice and Steamed Vegetables

Prep Time: 15 minutes: Cooking Time: 20 minutes: Serving Size: 4

Ingredients:

For the Tofu Teriyaki:

- 1 block (14 oz) extra-firm tofu, pressed and cubed
- 1/4 cup low-sodium soy sauce or tamari
- 2 tablespoons rice vinegar
- 2 tablespoons honey or maple syrup
- 2 cloves garlic, minced
- 1 teaspoon grated ginger
- 1 tablespoon cornstarch

- 2 tablespoons water
- Sesame seeds and sliced green onions for garnish (optional)

For the Brown Rice and Steamed Vegetables:

- 1 cup brown rice
- 2 cups water or vegetable broth
- Assorted vegetables for steaming (such as broccoli, carrots, and bell peppers)

Method of Preparation:

1. In a bowl, whisk together soy sauce, rice vinegar, honey or maple syrup, minced garlic, and grated ginger to make the teriyaki sauce.
2. In a separate small bowl, mix together cornstarch and water to make a slurry.
3. Heat a non-stick skillet over medium-high heat. Add cubed tofu and cook until golden brown on all sides.
4. Pour the teriyaki sauce over the tofu in the skillet. Add the cornstarch slurry and stir well to combine. Cook for 2-3 minutes, or until the sauce thickens and coats the tofu.
5. Meanwhile, cook brown rice according to package instructions.
6. Steam assorted vegetables until tender-crisp.
7. Serve tofu teriyaki over cooked brown rice, with steamed vegetables on the side. Garnish with sesame seeds and sliced green onions, if desired.

Nutritional Value (per serving): Calories: 350, Total Fat: 8g, Saturated Fat: 1g, Cholesterol: 0mg, Sodium: 550mg, Total Carbohydrates: 60g, Dietary Fiber: 8g, Sugars: 10g, Protein: 15g

Turkey Chili with Kidney Beans and Brown Rice

Prep Time: 15 minutes: Cooking Time: 30 minutes; Serving Size: 6

Ingredients:

- 1 lb ground turkey
- 1 tablespoon olive oil
- 1 onion, diced
- 2 cloves garlic, minced
- 1 bell pepper, diced
- 1 can (15 oz) diced tomatoes
- 1 can (15 oz) kidney beans, drained and rinsed
- 1 cup corn kernels (fresh or frozen)
- 2 tablespoons chili powder
- 1 teaspoon ground cumin
- Salt and pepper to taste
- Cooked brown rice, for serving
- Optional toppings: shredded cheese, diced avocado, chopped cilantro, sour cream

Method of Preparation:

1. In a large pot, heat olive oil over medium heat. Add diced onion, minced garlic, and diced bell pepper. Sauté until softened, about 5 minutes.

2. Add ground turkey to the pot. Cook until browned, breaking it up with a spoon as it cooks.

3. Stir in diced tomatoes, kidney beans, corn kernels, chili powder, ground cumin, salt, and pepper. Bring to a simmer.

4. Cover and cook for 20-25 minutes, stirring occasionally, until the chili has thickened and flavors have melded.

5. Serve turkey chili hot over cooked brown rice. Top with optional toppings such as shredded cheese, diced avocado, chopped cilantro, and sour cream.

Nutritional Value (per serving): Calories: 350, Total Fat: 10g, Saturated Fat: 2.5g, Cholesterol: 60mg, Sodium: 450mg, Total Carbohydrates: 40g, Dietary Fiber: 9g, Sugars: 6g, Protein: 25g

Chicken Breast with Caprese Salad and Whole-Wheat Couscous

Prep Time: 15 minutes: Cooking Time: 15 minutes: Serving Size: 4

Ingredients:

For the Chicken:

- 4 boneless, skinless chicken breasts
- 1 tablespoon olive oil
- 2 cloves garlic, minced
- 1 teaspoon dried oregano
- Salt and pepper to taste

For the Caprese Salad:

- 2 large tomatoes, sliced
- 1 ball fresh mozzarella cheese, sliced
- Fresh basil leaves
- Balsamic glaze (optional)
- Salt and pepper to taste

For the Whole-Wheat Couscous:

- 1 cup whole-wheat couscous
- 1 1/4 cups water or low-sodium chicken broth
- 1 tablespoon olive oil

Method of Preparation:

1. Preheat grill or grill pan over medium-high heat.
2. Season chicken breasts with olive oil, minced garlic, dried oregano, salt, and pepper.
3. Grill chicken breasts for 6-7 minutes per side, or until cooked through and no longer pink in the center.
4. While the chicken is cooking, prepare the caprese salad by layering sliced tomatoes, sliced fresh mozzarella, and fresh basil leaves on a serving platter. Drizzle with balsamic glaze, if desired. Season with salt and pepper to taste.
5. In a saucepan, bring water or chicken broth to a boil. Stir in whole-wheat couscous and olive oil. Remove from heat, cover, and let stand for 5 minutes. Fluff with a fork before serving.
6. Serve grilled chicken breasts with caprese salad and whole-wheat couscous on the side.

Nutritional Value (per serving): Calories: 380, Total Fat: 15g, Saturated Fat: 5g, Cholesterol: 80mg, Sodium: 450mg, Total Carbohydrates: 25g

Dietary Fiber: 4g

Sugars: 3g

Protein: 35g

Vegetarian Chili with Butternut Squash and Black Beans

Prep Time: 15 minutes: Cooking Time: 45 minutes: Serving Size: 6

Ingredients:

- 1 tablespoon olive oil
- 1 onion, diced
- 2 cloves garlic, minced
- 2 cups diced butternut squash
- 1 bell pepper, diced
- 1 can (15 oz) black beans, drained and rinsed
- 1 can (15 oz) diced tomatoes
- 2 cups vegetable broth
- 1 tablespoon chili powder
- 1 teaspoon ground cumin
- 1/2 teaspoon smoked paprika
- Salt and pepper to taste
- Fresh cilantro, chopped (for garnish)
- Optional toppings: shredded cheese, diced avocado, sour cream

Method of Preparation:

1. In a large pot, heat olive oil over medium heat. Add diced onion and minced garlic. Sauté until softened, about 5 minutes.
2. Add diced butternut squash and diced bell pepper to the pot. Cook for another 5 minutes, stirring occasionally.
3. Stir in drained and rinsed black beans, diced tomatoes (with juices), vegetable broth, chili powder, ground cumin, smoked paprika, salt, and pepper.

4. Bring the chili to a simmer, then reduce heat to low. Cover and cook for 30-35 minutes, or until the butternut squash is tender and flavors have melded.

5. Serve vegetarian chili hot, garnished with chopped fresh cilantro and optional toppings such as shredded cheese, diced avocado, and sour cream.

Nutritional Value (per serving): Calories: 250, Total Fat: 5g, Saturated Fat: 1g, Cholesterol: 0mg, Sodium: 450mg, Total Carbohydrates: 45g, Dietary Fiber: 12g, Sugars: 8g, Protein: 10g

Baked Tofu with Peanut Sauce and Stir-Fried Vegetables

Prep Time: 15 minutes: Cooking Time: 25 minutes: Serving Size: 4

Ingredients:

For the Baked Tofu:

- 1 block (14 oz) extra-firm tofu, pressed and sliced into cubes
- 2 tablespoons soy sauce or tamari
- 1 tablespoon sesame oil
- 1 tablespoon cornstarch
- Cooking spray

For the Peanut Sauce:

- 1/4 cup natural peanut butter
- 2 tablespoons soy sauce or tamari
- 1 tablespoon maple syrup or honey
- 1 tablespoon rice vinegar
- 1 clove garlic, minced
- 1 teaspoon grated ginger
- Water (as needed to thin out the sauce)

For the Stir-Fried Vegetables:

- 1 tablespoon olive oil
- 2 cups mixed vegetables (such as bell peppers, broccoli, carrots, and snap peas), sliced
- 2 cloves garlic, minced
- Salt and pepper to taste

Method of Preparation:

1. Preheat oven to 400°F (200°C). Line a baking sheet with parchment paper and lightly grease with cooking spray.

2. In a bowl, whisk together soy sauce, sesame oil, and cornstarch. Add cubed tofu and toss to coat. Arrange tofu in a single layer on the prepared baking sheet.

3. Bake tofu in the preheated oven for 20-25 minutes, flipping halfway through, until crispy and golden brown.

4. While the tofu is baking, prepare the peanut sauce. In a small saucepan, combine peanut butter, soy sauce, maple syrup or honey, rice vinegar, minced garlic, and grated ginger. Heat over low heat, stirring constantly, until smooth and well combined. If the sauce is too thick, thin it out with water to reach the desired consistency.

5. In a large skillet or wok, heat olive oil over medium-high heat. Add minced garlic and stir-fry for 1 minute, until fragrant.

6. Add sliced mixed vegetables to the skillet and stir-fry for 5-7 minutes, or until tender-crisp. Season with salt and pepper to taste.

7. Serve baked tofu with peanut sauce drizzled on top, alongside stir-fried vegetables.

Nutritional Value (per serving): Calories: 350, Total Fat: 20g, Saturated Fat: 3g, Cholesterol: 0mg, Sodium: 600mg, Total Carbohydrates: 25g, Dietary Fiber: 6g, Sugars: 8g

Protein: 20g

White Bean Soup with Kale and Whole-Wheat Toast

Prep Time: 15 minutes: Cooking Time: 30 minutes: Serving Size: 4

Ingredients:

- 1 tablespoon olive oil
- 1 onion, diced
- 2 cloves garlic, minced
- 2 carrots, diced
- 2 stalks celery, diced
- 4 cups vegetable broth
- 2 cans (15 oz each) white beans, drained and rinsed
- 2 cups chopped kale leaves
- 1 teaspoon dried thyme
- Salt and pepper to taste
- Whole-wheat bread slices, toasted (for serving)

Method of Preparation:

1. In a large pot, heat olive oil over medium heat. Add diced onion, minced garlic, diced carrots, and diced celery. Sauté until vegetables are softened, about 5 minutes.
2. Add vegetable broth to the pot and bring to a simmer.
3. Stir in drained and rinsed white beans, chopped kale leaves, and dried thyme. Season with salt and pepper to taste.

4. Simmer the soup for 15-20 minutes, or until the vegetables are tender and the flavors have melded.

5. Serve hot white bean soup with toasted whole-wheat bread slices on the side.

Nutritional Value (per serving): Calories: 300, Total Fat: 4g, Saturated Fat: 0.5g, Cholesterol: 0mg, Sodium: 700mg, Total Carbohydrates: 50g, Dietary Fiber: 12g, Sugars: 5g, Protein: 15g

Flank Steak Fajitas with Whole-Wheat Tortillas and Grilled Peppers

Prep Time: 20 minutes: Cooking Time: 15 minutes: Serving Size: 4

Ingredients:

For the Flank Steak:

- 1 lb flank steak
- 2 tablespoons olive oil
- 1 lime, juiced
- 2 cloves garlic, minced
- 1 teaspoon ground cumin
- 1 teaspoon chili powder
- Salt and pepper to taste

For the Grilled Peppers:

- 2 bell peppers (any color), sliced
- 1 onion, sliced
- 1 tablespoon olive oil
- Salt and pepper to taste

For Serving:

- 8 whole-wheat tortillas

- Optional toppings: salsa, guacamole, shredded cheese, sour cream

Method of Preparation:

1. In a bowl, whisk together olive oil, lime juice, minced garlic, ground cumin, chili powder, salt, and pepper to make the marinade for the flank steak.
2. Place flank steak in a shallow dish and pour the marinade over it. Allow the steak to marinate for at least 15 minutes, or up to 1 hour.
3. Preheat grill or grill pan over medium-high heat. Remove steak from marinade and discard excess marinade.
4. Grill flank steak for 4-6 minutes per side, or until desired level of doneness is reached. Remove from heat and let it rest for 5 minutes before slicing thinly against the grain.
5. Meanwhile, toss sliced bell peppers and onions with olive oil, salt, and pepper. Grill vegetables in a grill basket or on skewers until tender and slightly charred.
6. Warm whole-wheat tortillas on the grill for a few seconds on each side.
7. Serve sliced flank steak and grilled peppers and onions with warm whole-wheat tortillas and optional toppings.

Nutritional Value (per serving): Calories: 400, Total Fat: 15g, Saturated Fat: 3.5g, Cholesterol: 50mg, Sodium: 500mg, Total Carbohydrates: 40g, Dietary Fiber: 6g, Sugars: 5g, Protein: 25g

Chicken Stir-Fry with Snow Peas, Carrots, and Cashews

Prep Time: 15 minutes}: Cooking Time: 15 minutes: Serving Size: 4

Ingredients:

- 1 lb boneless, skinless chicken breasts, thinly sliced
- 2 tablespoons soy sauce or tamari
- 1 tablespoon cornstarch
- 2 tablespoons olive oil
- 2 cloves garlic, minced
- 1 teaspoon grated ginger
- 1 cup snow peas
- 1 cup sliced carrots
- 1/2 cup unsalted cashews
- Salt and pepper to taste
- Cooked brown rice, for serving

Method of Preparation:

1. In a bowl, whisk together soy sauce or tamari and cornstarch. Add sliced chicken breast to the bowl and toss to coat.
2. Heat olive oil in a large skillet or wok over medium-high heat. Add minced garlic and grated ginger, Stir-fry garlic and ginger for about 30 seconds until fragrant.
3. Add the coated chicken slices to the skillet and stir-fry for 5-6 minutes until cooked through and lightly browned.
4. Add snow peas and sliced carrots to the skillet, and continue to stir-fry for an additional 2-3 minutes until vegetables are tender-crisp.
5. Stir in unsalted cashews and cook for another minute.
6. Season the stir-fry with salt and pepper to taste.
7. Serve the chicken stir-fry hot over cooked brown rice.

Nutritional Value (per serving): Calories: 380, Total Fat: 18g, Saturated Fat: 3g, Cholesterol: 70mg, Sodium: 600mg, Total Carbohydrates: 20g, Dietary Fiber: 4g, Sugars: 5g, Protein: 35g

CHAPTER 4
Wholesome Side Dishes

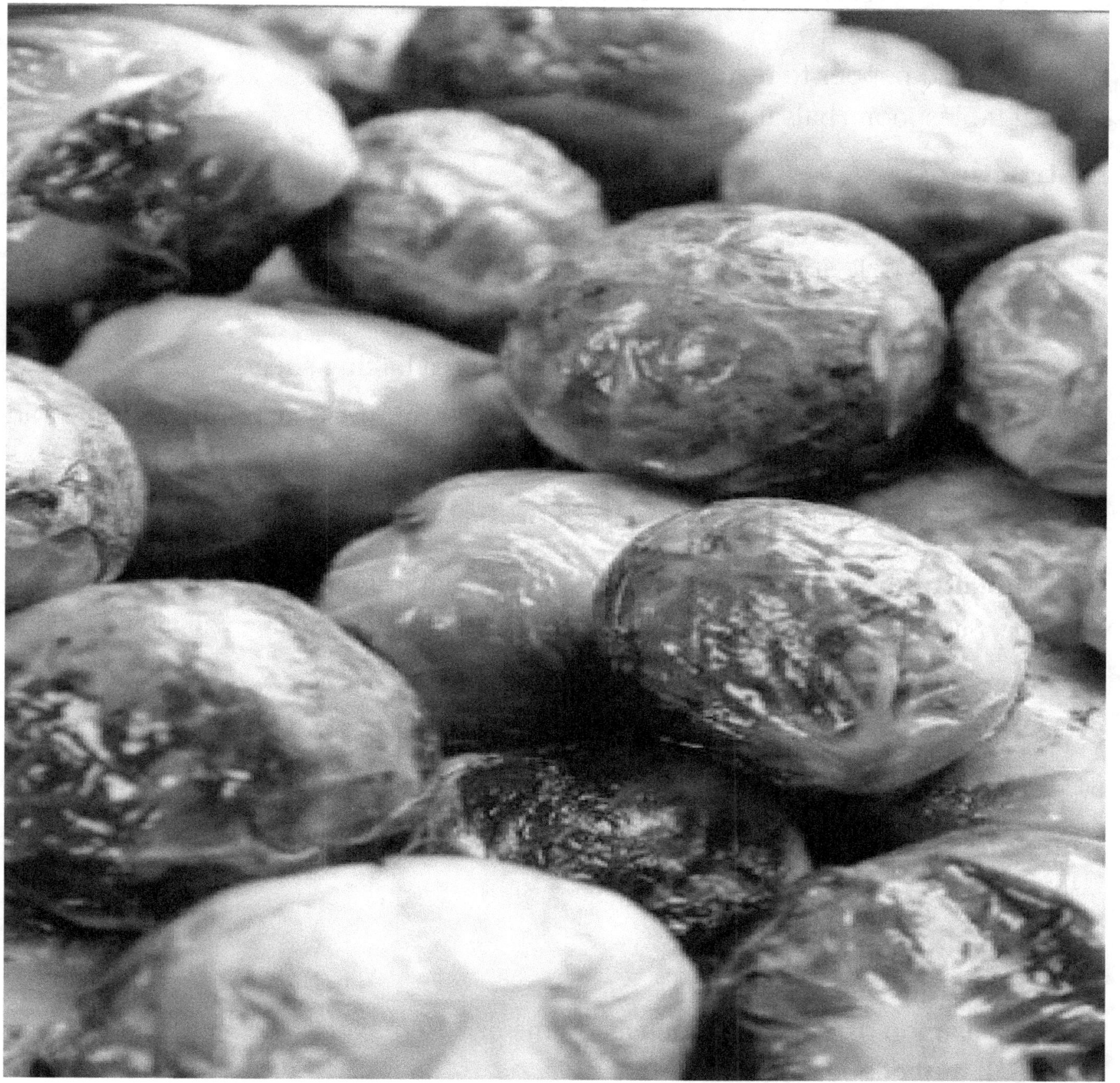

Balsamic Glazed Brussels Sprouts:

Prep Time: 10 minutes: Cooking Time: 25 minutes: Serving Size: 1 cup

Ingredients:

- 2 cups Brussels sprouts, trimmed and halved
- 1 tablespoon olive oil
- Salt and pepper to taste
- 2 tablespoons balsamic glaze

Instructions:

1. Preheat the oven to 400°F (200°C).
2. Toss Brussels sprouts with olive oil, salt, and pepper in a bowl until evenly coated.
3. Spread Brussels sprouts in a single layer on a baking sheet.
4. Roast in the preheated oven for 20-25 minutes, or until tender and caramelized, stirring halfway through.
5. Drizzle balsamic glaze over roasted Brussels sprouts before serving.

Nutritional Information (per serving): Calories: 120, Protein: 3g, Carbohydrates: 18g, Fiber: 6g, Sugar: 6g, Fat: 5g, Saturated Fat: 1g, Cholesterol: 0mg, Sodium: 30mg, Potassium: 400mg

Sauteed Green Beans with Garlic and Herbs:

Prep Time: 10 minutes: Cooking Time: 10 minutes: Serving Size: 1 cup

Ingredients:

- 2 cups green beans, trimmed
- 1 tablespoon olive oil
- 2 garlic cloves, minced
- 1 teaspoon dried herbs (such as thyme or rosemary)
- Salt and pepper to taste

- Lemon wedges for serving

Instructions:

1. Heat olive oil in a skillet over medium heat.
2. Add minced garlic and cook for 1 minute, until fragrant.
3. Add green beans to the skillet and sauté for 5-7 minutes, or until tender-crisp.
4. Sprinkle dried herbs over the green beans and toss to combine.
5. Season with salt and pepper to taste.
6. Serve hot with lemon wedges on the side.

Nutritional Information (per serving): Calories: 80, Protein: 2g, Carbohydrates: 8g, Fiber: 3g, Sugar: 2g, Fat: 5g, Saturated Fat: 1g, Cholesterol: 0mg, Sodium: 10mg, Potassium: 250mg

Creamy Cauliflower Mash with Parmesan Cheese:

Prep Time: 10 minutes: Cooking Time: 20 minutes: Serving Size: 1 cup

Ingredients:

- 1 medium head cauliflower, cut into florets
- 2 garlic cloves, peeled
- 2 tablespoons unsalted butter
- 1/4 cup grated Parmesan cheese
- Salt and pepper to taste
- Chopped fresh parsley for garnish

Instructions:

1. Place cauliflower florets and garlic cloves in a pot of boiling water. Cook until cauliflower is fork-tender, about 10-12 minutes.
2. Drain the cooked cauliflower and garlic cloves.

3. Transfer them to a food processor.
4. Add unsalted butter and grated Parmesan cheese to the food processor.
5. Pulse until cauliflower is smooth and creamy.
6. Season with salt and pepper to taste.
7. Transfer the creamy cauliflower mash to a serving dish.
8. Garnish with chopped fresh parsley before serving.

Nutritional Information (per serving): Calories: 120, Protein: 5g, Carbohydrates: 10g, Fiber: 4g, Sugar: 4g, Fat: 7g, Saturated Fat: 4g, Cholesterol: 20mg, Sodium: 150mg, Potassium: 500mg

Quinoa Salad with Chopped Vegetables and Vinaigrette:

Prep Time: 15 minutes: Cooking Time: 15 minutes: Serving Size: 1 cup

Ingredients:

- 1/2 cup quinoa, rinsed
- 1 cup water or vegetable broth
- 1 cup mixed chopped vegetables (such as bell peppers, cucumbers, cherry tomatoes)
- 2 tablespoons chopped fresh parsley
- 2 tablespoons olive oil
- 1 tablespoon balsamic vinegar
- 1 teaspoon Dijon mustard
- Salt and pepper to taste

Instructions:

1. In a pot, combine quinoa and water or vegetable broth.
2. Bring to a boil, then reduce heat to low. Cover and simmer for 15 minutes, or until quinoa is cooked and liquid is absorbed.
3. Fluff the cooked quinoa with a fork and let it cool.

4. In a large bowl, combine cooked quinoa, chopped vegetables, and chopped fresh parsley.
5. In a small bowl, whisk together olive oil, balsamic vinegar, Dijon mustard, salt, and pepper to make the vinaigrette.
6. Pour the vinaigrette over the quinoa salad and toss to coat everything evenly.
7. Serve chilled or at room temperature.

Nutritional Information (per serving): Calories: 200, Protein: 5g, Carbohydrates: 25g, Fiber: 4g, Sugar: 2g, Fat: 9g, Saturated Fat: 1g, Cholesterol: 0mg, Sodium: 100mg, Potassium: 250mg

Grilled Zucchini with Lemon and Olive Oil:

Prep Time: 10 minutes: Cooking Time: 10 minutes: Serving Size: 1 zucchini

Ingredients:

- 1 medium zucchini, sliced lengthwise into 1/4-inch-thick strips
- 1 tablespoon olive oil
- Zest and juice of 1 lemon
- Salt and pepper to taste
- Fresh chopped herbs (such as parsley or basil) for garnish

Instructions:

1. Preheat grill to medium-high heat.

2. In a bowl, toss zucchini strips with olive oil, lemon zest, lemon juice, salt, and pepper until evenly coated.

3. Place zucchini strips on the preheated grill and cook for 3-4 minutes per side, or until tender and grill marks appear.

4. Remove from the grill and transfer to a serving platter.

5. Garnish with fresh chopped herbs before serving.

Nutritional Information (per serving): Calories: 80, Protein: 2g, Carbohydrates: 5g, Fiber: 2g, Sugar: 2g, Fat: 6g, Saturated Fat: 1g, Cholesterol: 0mg, Sodium: 10mg, Potassium: 300mg

Baked Sweet Potato Wedges:

Prep Time: 10 minutes: Cooking Time: 25 minutes: Serving Size: 1 potato (about 1 cup)

Ingredients:

- 1 large sweet potato, scrubbed and cut into wedges
- 1 tablespoon olive oil
- 1 teaspoon paprika
- 1/2 teaspoon garlic powder
- 1/2 teaspoon onion powder
- Salt and pepper to taste

Instructions:

1. Preheat the oven to 425°F (220°C). Line a baking sheet with parchment paper.
2. In a bowl, toss sweet potato wedges with olive oil, paprika, garlic powder, onion powder, salt, and pepper until evenly coated.
3. Arrange sweet potato wedges in a single layer on the prepared baking sheet.
4. Bake in the preheated oven for 20-25 minutes, flipping halfway through, or until tender and golden brown.
5. Remove from the oven and let them cool for a few minutes before serving.

Nutritional Information (per serving): Calories: 120, Protein: 2g, Carbohydrates: 20g, Fiber: 3g, Sugar: 4g, Fat: 4g, Saturated Fat: 1g, Cholesterol: 0mg, Sodium: 150mg, Potassium: 400mg

Marinated Artichoke Hearts:

Prep Time: 5 minutes: Marinating Time: 1 hour: Serving Size: 1/2 cup

Ingredients:

- 1 (14 oz) can artichoke hearts, drained and quartered
- 2 tablespoons olive oil
- 1 tablespoon lemon juice
- 2 garlic cloves, minced
- 1 teaspoon dried oregano
- Salt and pepper to taste

Instructions:

1. In a bowl, whisk together olive oil, lemon juice, minced garlic, dried oregano, salt, and pepper to make the marinade.
2. Add drained and quartered artichoke hearts to the marinade.
3. Toss to coat artichoke hearts evenly with the marinade.
4. Cover and refrigerate for at least 1 hour to allow the flavors to meld.
5. Serve marinated artichoke hearts chilled or at room temperature.

Nutritional Information (per serving): Calories: 100, Protein: 2g

Carbohydrates: 5g, Fiber: 2g, Sugar: 0g, Fat: 8g, Saturated Fat: 1g

Cholesterol: 0mg, Sodium: 200mg, Potassium: 100mg

Coleslaw with Lightened Dressing:

Prep Time: 15 minutes: Chilling Time: 1 hour: Serving Size: 1 cup

Ingredients:

- 4 cups shredded cabbage (green or red cabbage or a mix)
- 1 large carrot, grated
- 1/4 cup plain Greek yogurt
- 2 tablespoons mayonnaise
- 1 tablespoon apple cider vinegar
- 1 teaspoon honey or maple syrup
- 1/2 teaspoon Dijon mustard
- Salt and pepper to taste
- Chopped fresh parsley or cilantro for garnish (optional)

Instructions:

1. In a large bowl, combine shredded cabbage and grated carrot.
2. In a small bowl, whisk together Greek yogurt, mayonnaise, apple cider vinegar, honey or maple syrup, Dijon mustard, salt, and pepper to make the dressing.
3. Pour the dressing over the shredded cabbage and grated carrot.
4. Toss to coat the coleslaw evenly with the dressing.
5. Cover and refrigerate for at least 1 hour before serving to allow the flavors to meld.
6. Garnish with chopped fresh parsley or cilantro before serving, if desired.

Nutritional Information (per serving): Calories: 80, Protein: 2g, Carbohydrates: 10g, Fiber: 3g, Sugar: 6g, Fat: 4g, Saturated Fat: 1g, Cholesterol: 5mg, Sodium: 120mg, Potassium: 250mg

Roasted Asparagus with Parmesan Cheese:

Prep Time: 10 minutes: Cooking Time: 15 minutes: Serving Size: 1 cup

Ingredients:

- 1 bunch asparagus, trimmed
- 1 tablespoon olive oil
- Salt and pepper to taste
- 2 tablespoons grated Parmesan cheese
- Lemon wedges for serving

Instructions:

1. Preheat the oven to 425°F (220°C).
2. Place trimmed asparagus on a baking sheet.
3. Drizzle olive oil over the asparagus and toss to coat evenly.
4. Season with salt and pepper to taste.
5. Roast in the preheated oven for 12-15 minutes, or until asparagus is tender and lightly browned.
6. Remove from the oven and sprinkle grated Parmesan cheese over the roasted asparagus.
7. Serve hot with lemon wedges on the side.

Nutritional Information (per serving): Calories: 60, Protein: 3g, Carbohydrates: 4g, Fiber: 2g, Sugar: 2g, Fat: 4g, Saturated Fat: 1g, Cholesterol: 5mg, Sodium: 100mg, Potassium: 250mg

Sauteed Mushrooms with Onions and Thyme:

Prep Time: 10 minutes: Cooking Time: 15 minutes: Serving Size: 1 cup

Ingredients:

- 2 cups sliced mushrooms (such as button or cremini)
- 1/2 cup sliced onion
- 2 garlic cloves, minced
- 1 tablespoon olive oil
- 1 teaspoon fresh thyme leaves
- Salt and pepper to taste

Instructions:

1. Heat olive oil in a skillet over medium heat.
2. Add sliced onions to the skillet and cook until softened, about 3-4 minutes.
3. Add minced garlic and cook for another 1-2 minutes, until fragrant.
4. Add sliced mushrooms to the skillet and cook, stirring occasionally, until mushrooms are golden brown and tender, about 8-10 minutes.
5. Stir in fresh thyme leaves and season with salt and pepper to taste.
6. Cook for an additional minute, then remove from heat.
7. Serve sautéed mushrooms and onions hot as a side dish or use as a topping for grilled meats or pasta.

Nutritional Information (per serving): Calories: 60, Protein: 3g, Carbohydrates: 6g, Fiber: 2g, Sugar: 3g, Fat: 4g, Saturated Fat: 0.5g, Cholesterol: 0mg, Sodium: 5mg, Potassium: 300mg

CHAPTER 5
Snack Attack Solutions

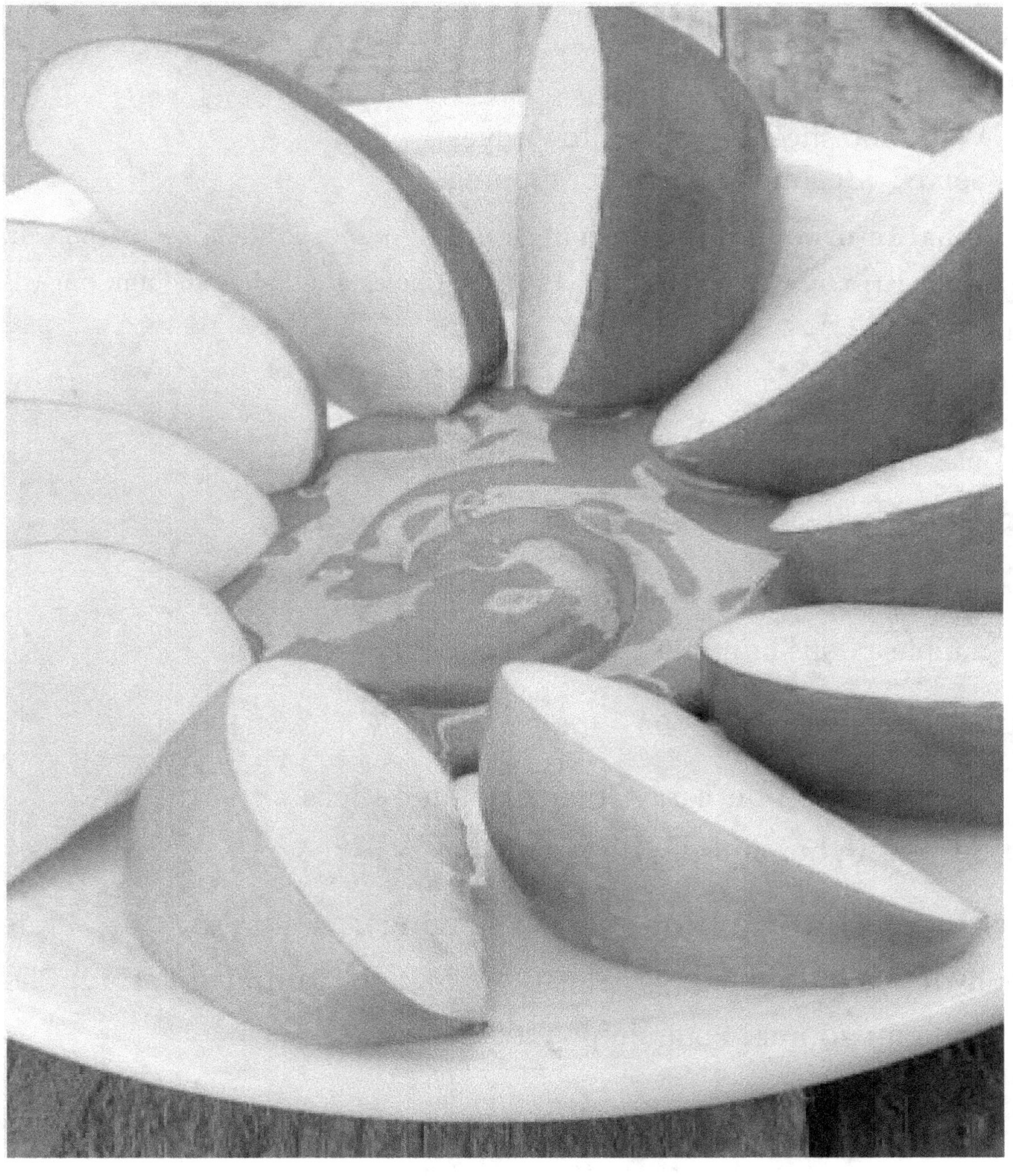

Apple Slices with Almond Butter

Prep Time: 5 minutes: Cooking Time: None: Serving Size: 1 apple, 2 tablespoons almond butter

Ingredients:

- 1 medium apple, sliced
- 2 tablespoons almond butter

Instructions:

1. Wash and slice the apple into wedges.
2. Serve with almond butter for dipping.

Nutritional Information (per serving): Calories: 200, Protein: 4g, Carbohydrates: 22g, Fiber: 5g, Sugar: 14g, Fat: 12g, Saturated Fat: 1g, Cholesterol: 0mg, Sodium: 0mg, Potassium: 195mg

Carrot Sticks with Hummus

Prep Time: 5 minutes: Cooking Time: None: Serving Size: 1

Ingredients:

- 2 medium carrots, cut into sticks
- 2 tablespoons hummus

Instructions:

1. Wash and peel the carrot, then cut it into sticks.
2. Serve with hummus for dipping.

Nutritional Information (per serving): Calories: 90, Protein: 3g, Carbohydrates: 10g, Fiber: 3g, Sugar: 3g, Fat: 5g, Saturated Fat: 1g, Cholesterol: 0mg, Sodium: 200mg, Potassium: 300mg

Edamame Pods

Prep Time: 5 minutes: Cooking Time: 5 minutes: Serving Size: 1 cup

Ingredients:

- 1 cup edamame pods (frozen, thawed)

Instructions:

1. Steam or boil the edamame pods until tender.
2. Drain and serve.

Nutritional Information (per serving): Calories: 120, Protein: 11g, Carbohydrates: 9g, Fiber: 4g, Sugar: 3g, Fat: 5g, Saturated Fat: 1g, Cholesterol: 0mg, Sodium: 5mg, Potassium: 375mg

Air-Popped Popcorn with Herbs and Spices

Prep Time: 5 minutes: Cooking Time: 5 minutes: Serving Size: 2 cups popped popcorn

Ingredients:

- 2 cups air-popped popcorn
- 1 teaspoon olive oil
- Herbs and spices to taste (such as garlic powder, paprika)

Instructions:

1. Pop the popcorn, drizzle with olive oil, and sprinkle with herbs and spices.
2. Toss to coat evenly and serve.

Nutritional Information (per serving): Calories: 80, Protein: 2g, Carbohydrates: 15g, Fiber: 3g, Sugar: 0g, Fat: 2g, Saturated Fat: 0g, Cholesterol: 0mg, Sodium: 0mg, Potassium: 60mg

Greek Yogurt with Chia Seeds and Berries

Prep Time: 5 minutes: Serving Size: 1

Ingredients:

- 1/2 cup Greek yogurt
- 1 tablespoon chia seeds
- 1/4 cup mixed berries (such as strawberries, blueberries, raspberries)

Instructions:

1. Mix Greek yogurt with chia seeds, then top with mixed berries.
2. Serve immediately.

Nutritional Information (per serving): Calories: 150, Protein: 12g, Carbohydrates: 12g, Fiber: 6g, Sugar: 4g, Fat: 6g, Saturated Fat: 1g, Cholesterol: 10mg, Sodium: 40mg, Potassium: 150mg

Cucumber Slices with Cottage Cheese and Dill

Prep Time: 5 minutes: Cooking Time: None: Serving Size: 1

Ingredients:

- 1/2 cucumber, sliced
- 1/4 cup cottage cheese
- Fresh dill for garnish (optional)

Instructions:

1. Wash and slice the cucumber.
2. Top cucumber slices with cottage cheese.
3. Garnish with fresh dill if desired.

Nutritional Information (per serving): Calories: 70, Protein: 7g, Carbohydrates: 5g, Fiber: 1g, Sugar: 3g, Fat: 2g, Saturated Fat: 1g, Cholesterol: 5mg, Sodium: 150mg, Potassium: 200mg

Bell Pepper Strips with Guacamole

Prep Time: 10 minutes: Cooking Time: None: Serving Size: 1

Ingredients:

- 1 medium bell pepper, sliced into strips
- 1 avocado
- 1 tablespoon lime juice
- Salt and pepper to taste

Instructions:

1. Wash and slice the bell pepper into strips.

2. Mash the avocado with lime juice, salt, and pepper to make guacamole.

3. Serve bell pepper strips with guacamole.

Nutritional Information (per serving): Calories: 130, Protein: 2g, Carbohydrates: 9g, Fiber: 5g, Sugar: 3g, Fat: 11g, Saturated Fat: 2g, Cholesterol: 0mg, Sodium: 10mg, Potassium: 400mg

Sliced Turkey Breast with Whole-Wheat Crackers

Prep Time: 5 minutes: Cooking Time: None: Serving Size: 3

Ingredients:

- 3 slices turkey breast (about 2 ounces)
- 6 whole-wheat crackers

Instructions:

1. Arrange turkey breast slices on a plate.

2. Serve with whole-wheat crackers.

Nutritional Information (per serving): Calories: 180, Protein: 18g, Carbohydrates: 15g, Fiber: 3g, Sugar: 1g, Fat: 6g, Saturated Fat: 1g, Cholesterol: 35mg, Sodium: 250mg, Potassium: 220mg

Handful of Mixed Nuts and Dried Cranberries

Prep Time: 2 minutes, Cooking Time: None, Serving Size: 1 handful (about 1/4 cup)

Ingredients:

- Assorted mixed nuts (such as almonds, walnuts, cashews)
- Dried cranberries

Instructions:

1. Combine a handful of mixed nuts with dried cranberries.
2. Enjoy as a satisfying snack.

Sweet Endings without the Sugar Spike

Prep Time: 10 minutes: Cooking Time: None: Serving Size: Varies

Ingredients:

- Fresh fruits (such as strawberries, blueberries, raspberries)
- Unsweetened whipped cream or Greek yogurt

Instructions:

1. Wash and prepare the fresh fruits.
2. Serve with a dollop of unsweetened whipped cream or Greek yogurt for dipping.
3. Enjoy as a guilt-free dessert option.

Spiced Pear with Ricotta Cheese

Prep Time: 5 minutes: Cooking Time: 5 minutes: Serving Size: 1

Ingredients:

- 1 ripe pear, halved and cored
- 2 tablespoons ricotta cheese
- Pinch of ground cinnamon
- Pinch of ground nutmeg
- 1 teaspoon honey (optional)

Instructions:

1. Place pear halves in a microwave-safe dish and sprinkle with cinnamon and nutmeg.
2. Microwave on high for 3-5 minutes, or until pear is tender.
3. Serve warm with a dollop of ricotta cheese on top.
4. Drizzle with honey if desired.

Nutritional Information (per serving): Calories: 150, Protein: 5g, Carbohydrates: 22g, Fiber: 5g, Sugar: 13g, Fat: 6g, Saturated Fat: 4g, Cholesterol: 20mg, Sodium: 40mg, Potassium: 210mg

Berry Bliss with Chia Seed Pudding

Prep Time: 5 minutes: Cooking Time: None (Refrigeration Time: 4 hours or overnight): Serving Size: 1/2 cup pudding, 1/4 cup mixed berries

Ingredients:

- 2 tablespoons chia seeds
- 1/2 cup unsweetened almond milk
- 1/2 teaspoon vanilla extract
- 1 teaspoon honey or maple syrup (optional)
- 1/4 cup mixed berries (such as strawberries, blueberries, raspberries)

Instructions:

1. In a bowl, whisk together chia seeds, almond milk, vanilla extract, and sweetener (if using).
2. Let the mixture sit for 5 minutes, then whisk again to break up any clumps.
3. Cover and refrigerate for at least 4 hours or overnight, until thickened.
4. Serve chia seed pudding with mixed berries on top.

Nutritional Information (per serving): Calories: 120, Protein: 3g, Carbohydrates: 14g, Fiber: 7g, Sugar: 5g, Fat: 6g, Saturated Fat: 1g, Cholesterol: 0mg, Sodium: 60mg, Potassium: 100mg

Citrus-Marinated Strawberries with Mint

Prep Time: 10 minutes: Marinating Time: 30 minutes: Serving Size: 1/2 cup

Ingredients:

- 1 cup strawberries, hulled and sliced
- Zest and juice of 1 lime or lemon
- 1 tablespoon honey or maple syrup (optional)
- Fresh mint leaves, chopped

Instructions:

1. In a bowl, combine sliced strawberries, lime or lemon zest, lime or lemon juice, and sweetener (if using).
2. Toss gently to coat the strawberries.
3. Cover and refrigerate for at least 30 minutes to allow flavors to meld.
4. Serve marinated strawberries topped with chopped mint leaves.

Nutritional Information (per serving): Calories: 50, Protein: 1g, Carbohydrate: 13g, Fiber: 3g, Sugar: 8g, Fat: 0g, Saturated Fat: 0g, Cholesterol: 0mg, Sodium: 0mg, Potassium: 220mg

Dark Chocolate Dipped Berries

Prep Time: 10 minutes: Cooking Time: 5 minutes: Serving Size: 1

Ingredients:

- 1/4 cup mixed berries (such as strawberries, blueberries, raspberries)
- 1 ounce dark chocolate (70% cocoa or higher), chopped

Instructions:

1. Wash and dry the berries, then set aside.
2. In a microwave-safe bowl, melt the dark chocolate in 30-second intervals, stirring in between until smooth.
3. Dip each berry halfway into the melted chocolate, then place on a parchment-lined baking sheet.
4. Refrigerate for 10-15 minutes, or until the chocolate sets.
5. Serve as a decadent snack or dessert.

Nutritional Information (per serving): Calories: 80, Protein: 1g, Carbohydrates: 12g, Fiber: 3g, Sugar: 7g, Fat: 4g, Saturated Fat: 2g, Cholesterol: 0mg, Sodium: 0mg, Potassium: 110mg

Roasted Figs with Goat Cheese

Prep Time: 5 minutes: Cooking Time: 10 minutes: Serving Size: 2

Ingredients:

1. 4 fresh figs, halved
2. 2 tablespoons honey
3. 2 tablespoons balsamic vinegar
4. 2 tablespoons crumbled goat cheese
5. Fresh thyme leaves for garnish (optional)

Instructions:

1. Preheat the oven to 400°F (200°C).

2. Place fig halves on a baking sheet, cut side up.

3. Drizzle honey and balsamic vinegar over the figs.

4. Roast in the preheated oven for 10 minutes, or until figs are tender.

5. Remove from the oven and let cool slightly.

6. Top each roasted fig half with crumbled goat cheese.

7. Garnish with fresh thyme leaves if desired.

8. Serve warm as a delicious appetizer or dessert.

Nutritional Information (per serving): Calories: 120, Protein: 2g, Carbohydrates: 18g, Fiber: 2g, Sugar: 15g, Fat: 5g, Saturated Fat: 3g, Cholesterol: 10mg, Sodium: 45mg, Potassium: 200mg

Cinnamon-Baked Apples with Walnuts

Prep Time: 10 minutes: Cooking Time: 30 minutes: Serving Size: 1 baked apple

Ingredients:

- 1 large apple (such as Granny Smith or Honeycrisp), cored
- 1 tablespoon melted coconut oil
- 1 tablespoon maple syrup or honey
- 1/2 teaspoon ground cinnamon
- 2 tablespoons chopped walnuts

Instructions:

1. Preheat the oven to 375°F (190°C).

2. Place the cored apple in a baking dish.

3. In a small bowl, mix together melted coconut oil, maple syrup or honey, and ground cinnamon.

4. Pour the mixture over the apple, making sure to coat it evenly.

5. Sprinkle chopped walnuts over the top of the apple.

6. Bake in the preheated oven for 25-30 minutes, or until the apple is tender.

7. Remove from the oven and let cool slightly before serving.

8. Serve warm as a comforting and nutritious dessert.

Nutritional Information (per serving): Calories: 220, Protein: 2g, Carbohydrates: 26g, Fiber: 5g, Sugar: 18g, Fat: 14g, Saturated Fat: 5g, Cholesterol: 0mg, Sodium: 0mg, Potassium: 210mg

Homemade Fruit Salad with a Squeeze of Lemon

Prep Time: 15 minutes: Serving Size: 1 cup

Ingredients:

- Assorted fresh fruits (such as strawberries, kiwi, pineapple, grapes, oranges)
- Juice of 1/2 lemon

Instructions:

1. Wash, peel, and chop the fruits into bite-sized pieces.

2. Place the chopped fruits in a bowl.

3. Squeeze fresh lemon juice over the fruits and toss gently to combine.

4. Serve immediately or refrigerate until ready to eat.

5. Enjoy this vibrant and refreshing fruit salad as a healthy snack or dessert option.

Nutritional Information (per serving): Varies depending on fruits

Poached Pears with Spices

Prep Time: 10 minutes: Cooking Time: 20 minutes: Serving Size: 1

Ingredients:

- 1 ripe pear, peeled and cored
- 1 cup water
- 1 tablespoon honey or maple syrup
- 1 cinnamon stick
- 2 whole cloves
- 1/2 teaspoon vanilla extract

Instructions:

1. In a saucepan, combine water, honey or maple syrup, cinnamon stick, cloves, and vanilla extract.
2. Bring the mixture to a gentle simmer over medium heat.
3. Add the peeled and cored pear to the simmering liquid.
4. Cover and let the pear poach for about 15-20 minutes, or until it's tender but not mushy.
5. Once poached, remove the pear from the liquid and let it cool slightly.
6. Serve the poached pear warm or chilled, drizzled with a little of the poaching liquid if desired.

Nutritional Information (per serving): Calories: 120; Protein: 1g; Carbohydrates: 30g; Fiber: 5g; Sugar: 20g, Fat: 0g; Saturated Fat: 0g

Cholesterol: 0mg, Sodium: 5mg, Potassium: 200mg

CHAPTER 6
Drinks and smoothies

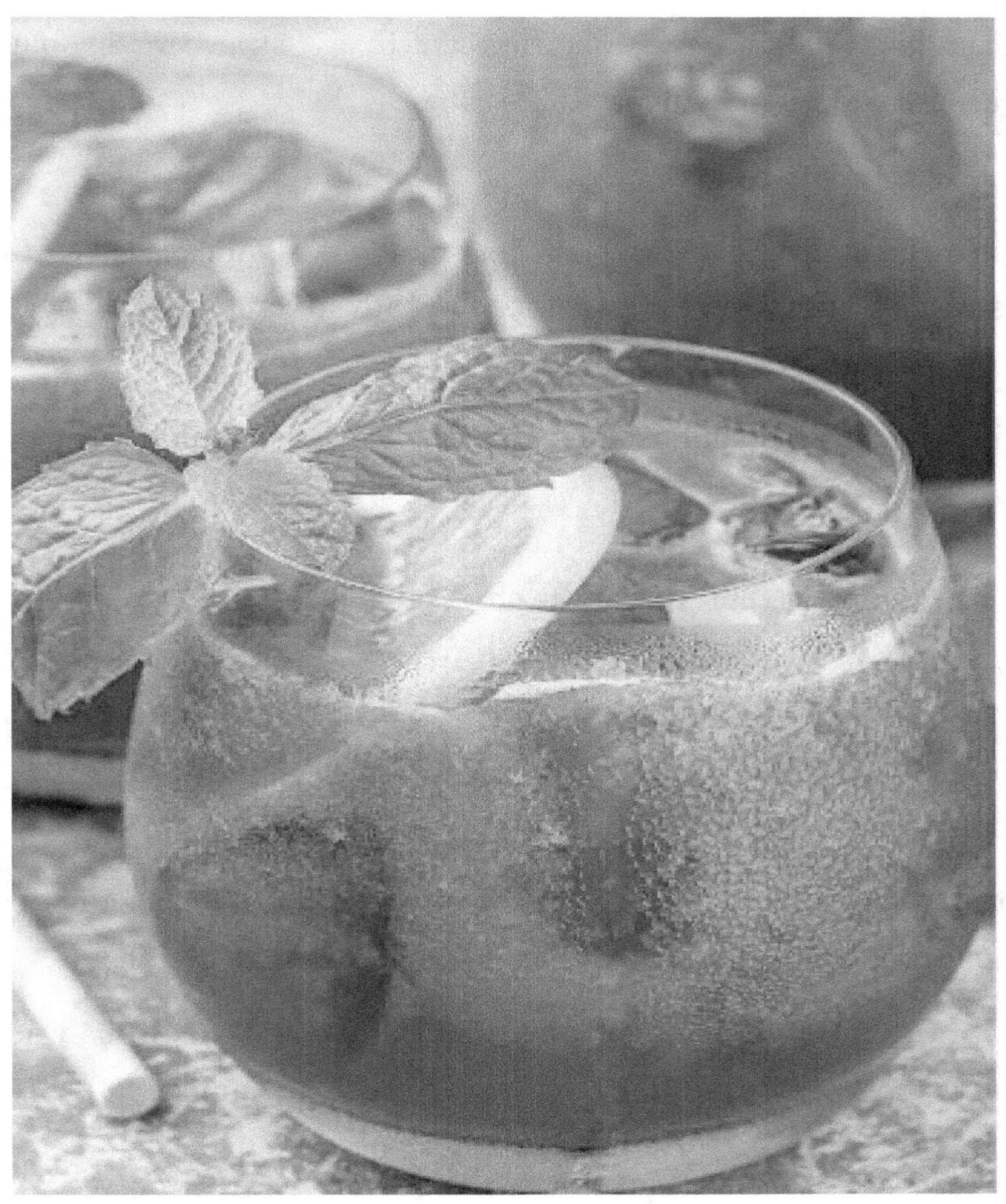

Sparkling Water with Berries and Mint:

Prep Time: 5 minutes

Ingredients:

- Sparkling water, mixed berries (such as strawberries, blueberries, raspberries), fresh mint leaves, ice cubes.

Method of Preparation:

1. In a glass, muddle a few berries and mint leaves. Add ice cubes, then pour sparkling water over the mixture. Stir gently to combine.

Nutritional Value: This drink is very low in calories and sugar, mainly providing hydration and a boost of antioxidants from the berries and mint.

Iced Green Tea with Lemon:

Prep Time: 5 minutes (plus time for tea to cool)

Ingredients:

- Green tea bags, water, lemon slices, ice cubes.

Method of Preparation:

1.Steep green tea bags in hot water for 3-5 minutes. Remove tea bags, add lemon slices, and let it cool to room temperature. Serve over ice.

Nutritional Value: Green tea is rich in antioxidants and has virtually no calories or sugar. Lemon adds a refreshing twist and a boost of vitamin C.

Sugar-Free Coffee with Cinnamon:

Prep Time: 5 minutes

Ingredients:

- Brewed coffee, ground cinnamon.

Method of Preparation:

1. Brew coffee as usual. Stir in ground cinnamon until well combined. Serve hot.

Nutritional Value: Coffee itself is very low in calories, but adding cinnamon can provide a touch of flavor without adding sugar. It also adds a negligible amount of calories.

Cucumber Mint Water:

Prep Time: 5 minutes

Ingredients:

- Cucumber slices, fresh mint leaves, water, ice cubes.

Method of Preparation:

1. In a pitcher, combine cucumber slices and mint leaves. Fill with water and refrigerate for at least 1 hour to allow flavors to infuse. Serve over ice.

Nutritional Value: Cucumber mint water is incredibly low in calories and sugar, making it an excellent choice for hydration. It also provides a refreshing and invigorating flavor.

Tomato and Basil Cooler:

Prep Time: 10 minutes

Ingredients:

- Tomato juice (unsweetened), fresh basil leaves, lemon juice, ice cubes.

Method of Preparation:

1. In a blender, combine tomato juice, fresh basil leaves, and lemon juice. Blend until smooth. Serve over ice.

Nutritional Value: This drink is rich in vitamins and minerals from the tomatoes and basil. It's low in calories and sugar, making it a refreshing and healthy choice.

Sugar-Free Flavored Water:

Prep Time: 5 minutes

Ingredients:

- Water, natural flavorings (such as sliced citrus fruits, berries, cucumber, herbs like mint or basil).

Method of Preparation:

1. Simply add your choice of natural flavorings to a pitcher of water. Let it infuse in the refrigerator for a few hours before serving over ice.

Nutritional Value: Flavored water is calorie-free and sugar-free, providing hydration with a hint of natural flavor.

Homemade Vegetable Juice:

Prep Time: 10 minutes

Ingredients:

- Assorted vegetables (such as carrots, celery, tomatoes, spinach), lemon juice, optional seasonings like black pepper or cayenne pepper.

Method of Preparation:

1. Juice the vegetables using a juicer. Mix the vegetable juice with a squeeze of lemon juice and any optional seasonings to taste.

Nutritional Value: Vegetable juice is rich in vitamins, minerals, and antioxidants. It's low in calories and sugar, making it a healthy choice for hydration and nutrition.

Sparkling Cranberry Limeade:

Prep Time: 5 minutes

Ingredients:

- Sparkling water, unsweetened cranberry juice, fresh lime juice, ice cubes.

Method of Preparation:

1. In a glass, combine sparkling water, unsweetened cranberry juice, and fresh lime juice. Stir well and add ice cubes.

Nutritional Value: This drink is low in calories and sugar, with a tangy flavor from the cranberry and lime. It's refreshing and perfect for hot days.

Coconut Water:

Prep Time: 2 minutes

Ingredients:

- Coconut water.

Method of Preparation:

1. Simply pour chilled coconut water into a glass and serve.

Nutritional Value: Coconut water is naturally low in calories and sugar. It's also rich in electrolytes, making it a hydrating and refreshing beverage.

Spiced Apple Cider:

Prep Time: 10 minutes

Ingredients:

- Unsweetened apple cider, cinnamon sticks, cloves, star anise (optional).

Method of Preparation:

- In a saucepan, heat apple cider with cinnamon sticks, cloves, and star anise (if using) until warm. Strain and serve hot.

Nutritional Value: Apple cider is rich in vitamin C and antioxidants. This sugar-free version is warming and perfect for chilly days.

Kefir Smoothie:

Prep Time: 5 minutes

Ingredients:

- Plain kefir, mixed berries (such as strawberries, blueberries, raspberries), banana, spinach (optional), ice cubes.

Method of Preparation:

- Blend kefir, mixed berries, banana, and spinach (if using) until smooth. Add ice cubes and blend again until creamy.

Nutritional Value: Kefir is a fermented dairy product that is rich in probiotics. This smoothie is packed with vitamins, minerals, and gut-friendly bacteria. Adjust sweetness by choosing naturally sweet fruits.

Sugar-Free Protein Shake:

Prep Time: 5 minutes

Ingredients:

- Unsweetened almond milk or coconut milk, protein powder (unsweetened), almond butter (unsweetened), ice cubes.

Method of Preparation:

- Blend almond milk, protein powder, and almond butter until smooth. Add ice cubes and blend again until creamy.

Nutritional Value: This protein shake is high in protein and low in sugar. It's perfect for a post-workout refuel or a nutritious snack. Adjust sweetness by choosing flavored or unflavored protein powder.

Green Power Smoothie:

Prep Time: 5 minutes

Ingredients:

- Spinach, cucumber, avocado, almond milk, chia seeds.

Method of Preparation:

- Blend spinach, cucumber, avocado, almond milk, and chia seeds until smooth. Adjust the consistency by adding more almond milk if necessary.

Nutritional Value: This smoothie is packed with nutrients like vitamins, minerals, fiber, and healthy fats. It's low in sugar and provides a good dose of plant-based protein from the chia seeds.

Berry Blast Smoothie:

Prep Time: 5 minutes

Ingredients:

- Mixed berries (strawberries, blueberries, raspberries), Greek yogurt (unsweetened), spinach, almond milk.

Method of Preparation:

- Blend mixed berries, Greek yogurt, spinach, and almond milk until smooth. Add more almond milk if needed to reach desired consistency.

Nutritional Value: This smoothie is rich in antioxidants from the berries, calcium and protein from the Greek yogurt, and vitamins and minerals from the spinach. It's low in sugar and provides a refreshing burst of flavor.

Creamy Peanut Butter Banana Smoothie:

Prep Time: 5 minutes

Ingredients:

- Banana, natural peanut butter (unsweetened), Greek yogurt (unsweetened), almond milk.

Method of Preparation:

- Blend banana, peanut butter, Greek yogurt, and almond milk until smooth. Adjust sweetness by adding a natural sweetener like stevia or honey if desired.

Nutritional Value: This smoothie is a great source of potassium from the banana, healthy fats and protein from the peanut butter, and probiotics from the Greek yogurt. It's low in added sugar and provides sustained energy.

Tropical Paradise Smoothie:

Prep Time: 5 minutes

Ingredients:

- Mango, pineapple, spinach, coconut milk (unsweetened).

Method of Preparation:

- Blend mango, pineapple, spinach, and coconut milk until smooth. Adjust consistency with water if needed.

Nutritional Value: This smoothie is bursting with tropical flavors and provides a wealth of vitamins, minerals, and antioxidants from the fruits and spinach. It's naturally sweet and low in added sugar.

Cinnamon Apple Smoothie:

Prep Time: 5 minutes

Ingredients:

- Apple, cinnamon, Greek yogurt (unsweetened), almond milk.

Method of Preparation:

- Blend apple, cinnamon, Greek yogurt, and almond milk until smooth. Adjust sweetness with a natural sweetener if desired.

Nutritional Value: This smoothie is reminiscent of apple pie flavors and is rich in fiber, vitamins, and minerals from the apple. It's low in sugar and provides a satisfying and nutritious snack or breakfast option.

Chocolate Avocado Smoothie:

Prep Time: 5 minutes

Ingredients:

- Avocado, cocoa powder (unsweetened), spinach, almond milk, stevia (optional).

Method of Preparation:

- Blend avocado, cocoa powder, spinach, almond milk, and stevia (if using) until smooth. Adjust sweetness to taste.

Nutritional Value: This smoothie is creamy and indulgent, thanks to the avocado and cocoa powder. It's high in healthy fats, fiber, and antioxidants, and can satisfy chocolate cravings without added sugar.

Vanilla Almond Protein Smoothie:

Prep Time: 5 minutes

Ingredients:

- Almond milk, vanilla protein powder (unsweetened), almond butter (unsweetened), spinach.

Method of Preparation:

- Blend almond milk, protein powder, almond butter, and spinach until smooth. Adjust sweetness with a natural sweetener if desired.

Nutritional Value: This smoothie is rich in plant-based protein, healthy fats, vitamins, and minerals. It's low in sugar and provides a satisfying and nutritious option for post-workout recovery or a quick meal replacement.

Peachy Keen Smoothie:

Prep Time: 5 minutes

Ingredients:

- Peach, Greek yogurt (unsweetened), spinach, almond milk.

Method of Preparation:

- Blend peach, Greek yogurt, spinach, and almond milk until smooth. Adjust sweetness with a natural sweetener if desired.

Nutritional Value: This smoothie offers a delightful combination of sweet peach flavor, creamy texture from Greek yogurt, and the added nutrients from spinach. It's low in sugar and provides a good source of vitamins and minerals.

Blueberry Kale Smoothie:

Prep Time: 5 minutes

Ingredients:

- Blueberries, kale, Greek yogurt (unsweetened), almond milk.

Method of Preparation:

- Blend blueberries, kale, Greek yogurt, and almond milk until smooth. Adjust sweetness with a natural sweetener if needed.

Nutritional Value: Packed with antioxidants from blueberries and kale, this smoothie is a powerhouse of nutrients. The Greek yogurt adds creaminess and protein while almond milk provides a dairy-free base.

Carrot Ginger Juice:

Prep Time: 10 minutes

Ingredients:

- Carrots, ginger, lemon.

Method of Preparation:

- Juice carrots and ginger together, then squeeze lemon juice into the mixture. Stir well and serve over ice if desired.

Nutritional Value: This juice is rich in beta-carotene from carrots, anti-inflammatory properties from ginger, and a hint of citrusy flavor from lemon. It's low in calories and sugar, making it a refreshing and nutritious option.

Green Apple Kale Juice:

Prep Time: 10 minutes

Ingredients:

- Green apple, kale, celery, lemon.

Method of Preparation:

- Juice green apple, kale, and celery together, then squeeze lemon juice into the mixture. Stir well and serve over ice if desired.

Nutritional Value: This juice is packed with vitamins and minerals from the green apple, kale, and celery. It's low in calories and sugar, making it a nutrient-dense beverage.

Beetroot Berry Juice:

Prep Time: 10 minutes

Ingredients:

Beetroot, mixed berries (strawberries, blueberries, raspberries), lemon.

Method of Preparation:

- Juice beetroot and mixed berries together, then squeeze lemon juice into the mixture. Stir well and serve over ice if desired.

Nutritional Value: Beetroot provides antioxidants and nitrates, while mixed berries add a burst of flavor and additional antioxidants. This juice is low in calories and sugar, making it a healthy option.

Spinach Pineapple Juice:

Prep Time: 10 minutes

Ingredients:

- Spinach, pineapple, cucumber, lime.

Method of Preparation:

- Juice spinach, pineapple, and cucumber together, then squeeze lime juice into the mixture. Stir well and serve chilled.

Nutritional Value: Spinach is rich in vitamins and minerals, while pineapple adds sweetness and tanginess. This juice is low in calories and sugar, making it a nutritious choice.

Turmeric Carrot Juice:

Prep Time: 10 minutes

Ingredients:

- Carrots, turmeric, ginger, lemon.

Method of Preparation:

- Juice carrots, turmeric, and ginger together, then squeeze lemon juice into the mixture. Stir well and serve over ice if desired.

Nutritional Value: This juice offers anti-inflammatory benefits from turmeric and ginger, along with vitamins and minerals from carrots and lemon. It's low in calories and sugar, making it a healthful beverage option.

Orange Ginger Juice:

Prep Time: 10 minutes

Ingredients:

- Oranges, ginger, turmeric.

Method of Preparation:

- Juice oranges and ginger together, then add a pinch of turmeric. Stir well and serve chilled.

Nutritional Value: Oranges provide vitamin C, while ginger and turmeric offer anti-inflammatory properties. This juice is low in calories and sugar, making it a refreshing and nutritious choice.

Cranberry Cabbage Juice:

Prep Time: 10 minutes

Ingredients:

- Cranberries, red cabbage, cucumber, lemon.

Method of Preparation:

- Juice cranberries, red cabbage, and cucumber together, then squeeze lemon juice into the mixture. Stir well and serve over ice if desired.

Nutritional Value: Cranberries are rich in antioxidants, while red cabbage adds vitamins and minerals. This juice is low in calories and sugar, making it a vibrant and healthful beverage.

Watermelon Basil Juice:

Prep Time: 10 minutes

Ingredients:

- Watermelon, basil leaves, lime.

Method of Preparation:

- Blend watermelon and basil leaves together until smooth. Squeeze lime juice into the mixture and stir well. Serve chilled.

Nutritional Value: Watermelon is hydrating and low in calories, while basil adds a refreshing flavor. Lime juice adds a citrusy kick. This juice is naturally sweet and low in sugar, making it a delicious and nutritious option.

Pineapple Spinach Smoothie:

Prep Time: 5 minutes

Ingredients:

- Pineapple chunks, spinach, Greek yogurt (unsweetened), coconut water.

Method of Preparation:

- Blend pineapple chunks, spinach, Greek yogurt, and coconut water until smooth. Add more coconut water if needed to reach desired consistency.

Nutritional Value: This smoothie offers a tropical flavor from pineapple and hydrating properties from coconut water. Spinach adds nutrients like vitamins A and C, while Greek yogurt provides protein and creaminess. It's low in added sugar and high in vitamins and minerals.

Minty Mango Smoothie:

Prep Time: 5 minutes

Ingredients:

- Mango chunks, fresh mint leaves, plain yogurt (unsweetened), almond milk.

Method of Preparation:

- Blend mango chunks, fresh mint leaves, plain yogurt, and almond milk until smooth. Adjust sweetness with a natural sweetener if desired.

Nutritional Value: This smoothie offers a refreshing blend of sweet mango and cooling mint flavors. It's rich in vitamins A and C from mango and provides probiotics from yogurt. Almond milk adds creaminess without adding sugar.

Kiwi Berry Blast Smoothie:

Prep Time: 5 minutes

Ingredients:

- Kiwi, mixed berries (strawberries, blueberries, raspberries), spinach, coconut water.

Method of Preparation:

- Blend kiwi, mixed berries, spinach, and coconut water until smooth. Add more coconut water if needed for desired consistency.

Nutritional Value: This smoothie is packed with antioxidants from berries, vitamin C from kiwi, and vitamins A and K from spinach. Coconut water provides hydration and natural sweetness. It's low in sugar and high in nutrients.

Creamy Avocado Banana Smoothie:

Prep Time: 5 minutes

Ingredients:

- Avocado, banana, plain Greek yogurt (unsweetened), almond milk.

Method of Preparation:

- Blend avocado, banana, Greek yogurt, and almond milk until smooth. Adjust sweetness with a natural sweetener if desired.

Nutritional Value: This smoothie is rich in healthy fats from avocado, potassium from banana, and protein from Greek yogurt. It's creamy and satisfying without added sugar, making it a nutritious breakfast or snack option.

Orange Carrot Ginger Juice:

Prep Time: 10 minutes

Ingredients:

- Oranges, carrots, ginger, turmeric.

Method of Preparation:

- Juice oranges, carrots, and ginger together, then add a pinch of turmeric. Stir well and serve chilled.

Nutritional Value: Oranges provide vitamin C, while carrots offer beta-carotene and ginger provides anti-inflammatory properties. Turmeric adds color and additional health benefits. This juice is low in calories and sugar, making it a refreshing and nutritious beverage.

Green Grape Kale Juice:

Prep Time: 10 minutes

Ingredients:

- Green grapes, kale, cucumber, lemon.

Method of Preparation:

- Juice green grapes, kale, and cucumber together, then squeeze lemon juice into the mixture. Stir well and serve over ice if desired.

Nutritional Value: Green grapes add sweetness and hydration, while kale and cucumber offer vitamins, minerals, and antioxidants. Lemon juice adds a citrusy kick. This juice is low in calories and sugar, making it a healthful option.

Strawberry Basil Lemonade:

Prep Time: 10 minutes

Ingredients:

- Strawberries, fresh basil leaves, lemon juice, water, stevia (optional).

Method of Preparation:

- Blend strawberries, basil leaves, lemon juice, and water until smooth. Adjust sweetness with stevia if desired. Serve over ice.

Nutritional Value: This refreshing drink combines the sweetness of strawberries with the herbaceous flavor of basil and the tartness of lemon. It's low in calories and sugar, making it a guilt-free treat.

Minty Watermelon Cucumber Cooler:

Prep Time: 10 minutes

Ingredients:

- Watermelon chunks, cucumber slices, fresh mint leaves, lime juice, sparkling water.

Method of Preparation:

In a blender, blend watermelon chunks, cucumber slices, fresh mint leaves, and lime juice until smooth. Pour the mixture into glasses and top with sparkling water. Stir gently and serve over ice.

Nutritional Value: This hydrating and refreshing drink combines the sweetness of watermelon with the crispness of cucumber and the coolness of mint. It's low in calories and sugar, making it perfect for staying refreshed on hot days.

Pomegranate Blueberry Smoothie:

Prep Time: 5 minutes

Ingredients:

- Pomegranate seeds, blueberries, Greek yogurt (unsweetened), almond milk.

Method of Preparation:

Blend pomegranate seeds, blueberries, Greek yogurt, and almond milk until smooth. Adjust sweetness with a natural sweetener if desired.

Nutritional Value: This smoothie is packed with antioxidants from pomegranate seeds and blueberries. Greek yogurt adds protein and creaminess while almond milk provides a dairy-free base. It's low in added sugar and high in vitamins and minerals.

Papaya Coconut Smoothie:

Prep Time: 5 minutes

Ingredients:

- Papaya chunks, coconut milk (unsweetened), plain yogurt (unsweetened), honey or stevia (optional).

Method of Preparation:

- Blend papaya chunks, coconut milk, plain yogurt, and honey or stevia (if using) until smooth. Adjust sweetness to taste.

Nutritional Value: This tropical smoothie offers a sweet and creamy flavor from papaya and coconut milk. Plain yogurt adds probiotics and protein, while honey or stevia can be used for sweetness without adding sugar.

Cherry Almond Smoothie:

Prep Time: 5 minutes

Ingredients:

- Cherries (pitted), almond butter (unsweetened), spinach, almond milk.

Method of Preparation:

- Blend cherries, almond butter, spinach, and almond milk until smooth. Adjust sweetness with a natural sweetener if desired.

Nutritional Value: Cherries provide antioxidants and a natural sweetness, while almond butter adds creaminess and healthy fats. Spinach adds nutrients without affecting the flavor. This smoothie is low in sugar and high in vitamins and minerals.

Raspberry Coconut Water Smoothie:

Prep Time: 5 minutes

Ingredients:

- Raspberries, coconut water, plain yogurt (unsweetened), chia seeds.

Method of Preparation:

- Blend raspberries, coconut water, plain yogurt, and chia seeds until smooth. Adjust sweetness with a natural sweetener if desired.

Nutritional Value: This refreshing smoothie combines the tartness of raspberries with the hydrating properties of coconut water. Plain yogurt adds creaminess and probiotics, while chia seeds offer omega-3 fatty acids and fiber.

Lemon Blueberry Kale Smoothie:

Prep Time: 5 minutes

Ingredients:

- Blueberries, kale, lemon juice, plain yogurt (unsweetened), almond milk.

Method of Preparation:

- Blend blueberries, kale, lemon juice, plain yogurt, and almond milk until smooth. Adjust sweetness with a natural sweetener if desired.

Nutritional Value: Blueberries provide antioxidants and sweetness, while kale adds vitamins and minerals. Lemon juice adds a tangy flavor, and almond milk provides creaminess. This smoothie is low in sugar and high in nutrients.

Banana Walnut Smoothie:

Prep Time: 5 minutes

Ingredients:

- Banana, walnuts, cinnamon, plain Greek yogurt (unsweetened), almond milk.

Method of Preparation:

- Blend banana, walnuts, cinnamon, plain Greek yogurt, and almond milk until smooth. Adjust sweetness with a natural sweetener if desired.

Nutritional Value: Bananas provide potassium and natural sweetness, while walnuts add omega-3 fatty acids and crunch. Cinnamon adds warmth and flavor, and Greek yogurt provides protein and creaminess. This smoothie is low in sugar and high in nutrients.

Mango Pineapple Coconut Smoothie:

Prep Time: 5 minutes

Ingredients:

- Mango chunks, pineapple chunks, coconut milk (unsweetened), plain yogurt (unsweetened).

Method of Preparation:

- Blend mango chunks, pineapple chunks, coconut milk, and plain yogurt until smooth. Adjust sweetness with a natural sweetener if desired.

Nutritional Value: This tropical smoothie offers a combination of sweet mango and pineapple flavors with creamy coconut milk. Plain yogurt adds probiotics and creaminess. It's low in sugar and high in vitamins and minerals.

Mixed Berry Protein Smoothie:

Prep Time: 5 minutes

Ingredients:

- Mixed berries (strawberries, blueberries, raspberries), protein powder (unsweetened), spinach, almond milk.

Method of Preparation:

- Blend mixed berries, protein powder, spinach, and almond milk until smooth. Adjust sweetness with a natural sweetener if desired.

Nutritional Value: This protein-packed smoothie offers a mix of antioxidants from berries, vitamins and minerals from spinach, and protein from protein powder. It's low in sugar and high in nutrients, making it a great post-workout snack or meal replacement.

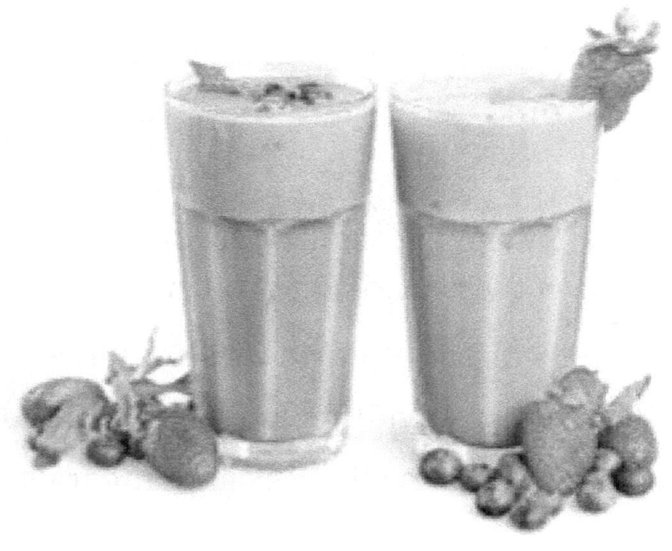

CHAPTER 7:

Meal Planning Made Easy

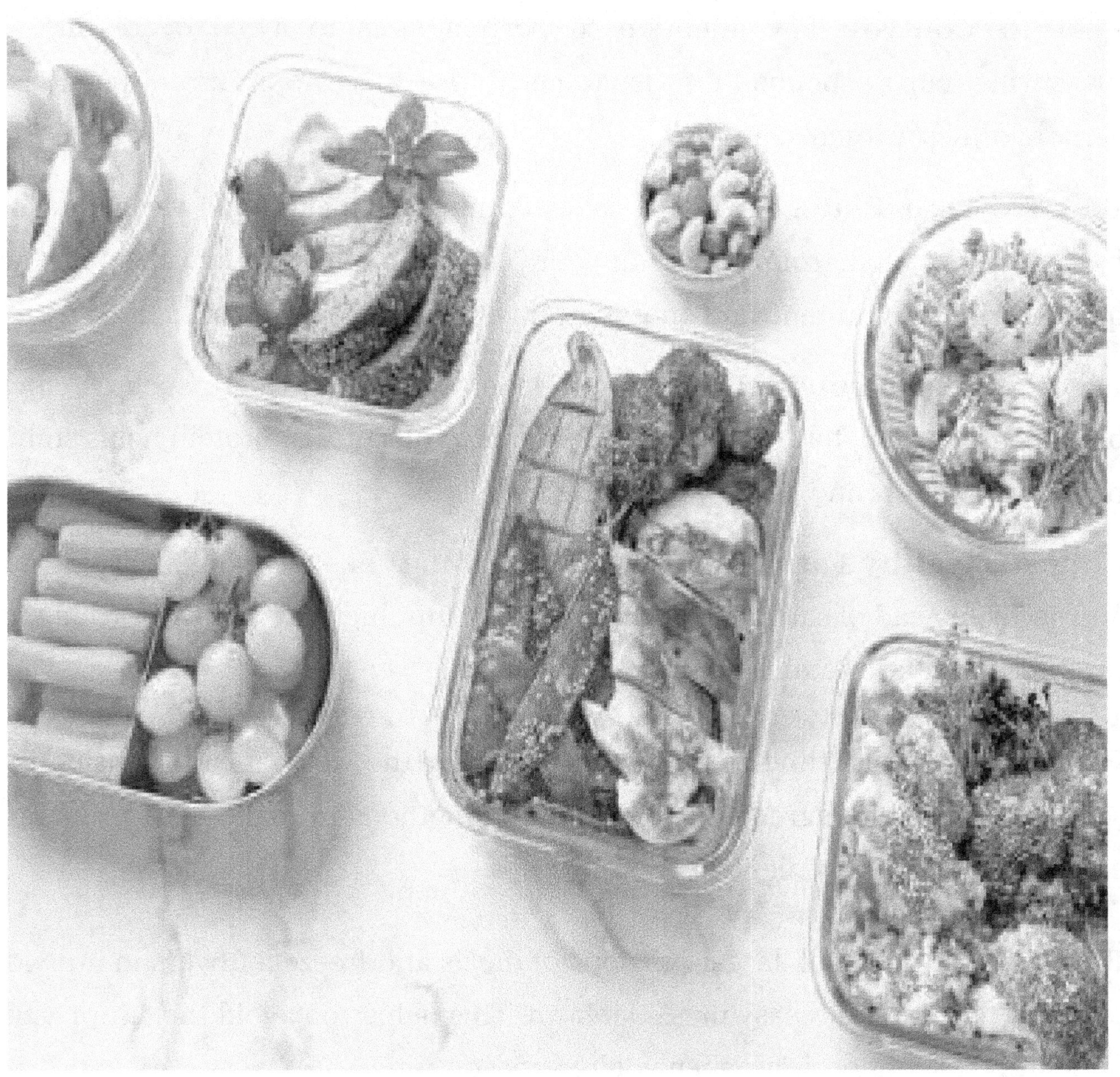

Bonus: Meal Planning Basics

Know Your Carbs: Be aware of the carbohydrate content in your meals as they affect blood sugar levels. Choose whole grains, fruits, vegetables, and legumes for healthier options.

Portion Control: Pay attention to portion sizes to avoid overeating. Use measuring cups, spoons, or visual cues to gauge appropriate portions of carbohydrates, proteins, and fats.

Balance Your Plate: Aim for a balanced meal by including a variety of foods from different food groups. Fill half your plate with non-starchy vegetables, one-quarter with lean protein, and one-quarter with whole grains or starchy vegetables.

Include Lean Proteins: Incorporate lean sources of protein such as chicken breast, turkey, fish, tofu, beans, and lentils into your meals. Protein helps stabilize blood sugar levels and keeps you feeling full.

Choose Healthy Fats: Opt for heart-healthy fats like olive oil, avocados, nuts, and seeds instead of saturated and trans fats. Limit high-fat foods like fried foods, processed meats, and full-fat dairy products.

Plan Ahead: Take time to plan your meals for the week ahead. Consider your schedule, available ingredients, and cooking methods to make meal preparation easier and more convenient.

Batch Cooking: Cook larger portions of meals and freeze leftovers in individual portions for quick and easy meals later on. This helps you avoid the temptation of unhealthy takeout options when you're short on time.

Read Food Labels: Pay attention to food labels and choose products with lower amounts of added sugars, sodium, and saturated fats. Look for whole, unprocessed foods whenever possible.

Stay Hydrated: Drink plenty of water throughout the day to stay hydrated and support overall health. Limit sugary drinks and opt for water, herbal teas, or infused water with lemon or cucumber for added flavor.

Listen to Your Body: Monitor your blood sugar levels regularly and pay attention to how different foods affect your body. Adjust your meal plan as needed based on your individual health goals and preferences.

Shopping for Diabetes-Friendly Ingredients

When shopping for diabetes-friendly ingredients, it's essential to make smart choices to support your health goals. Here are some tips for navigating the grocery store:

Focus on Whole Foods: Choose whole, unprocessed foods whenever possible. These include fresh fruits and vegetables, lean proteins, whole grains, and healthy fats.

Load Up on Non-Starchy Vegetables: Fill your cart with a variety of colorful vegetables such as leafy greens, broccoli, bell peppers, carrots, and tomatoes. These are low in calories and carbohydrates, high in fiber, and packed with essential vitamins and minerals.

Opt for Lean Proteins: Select lean cuts of meat such as skinless poultry, fish, and lean cuts of beef or pork. Incorporate plant-based protein sources like tofu, tempeh, beans, lentils, and legumes into your meals.

Choose Whole Grains: Look for whole grains like brown rice, quinoa, barley, oats, and whole wheat bread or pasta. These provide fiber, which helps regulate blood sugar levels and promotes digestive health.

Read Food Labels: Pay attention to food labels and ingredient lists. Look for products with minimal added sugars, sodium, and unhealthy fats. Aim for items with shorter ingredient lists and recognizable ingredients.

Limit Processed Foods: Minimize your intake of processed and packaged foods, which often contain added sugars, refined carbohydrates, and unhealthy fats. These can cause blood sugar spikes and contribute to weight gain.

Be Mindful of Portion Sizes: Keep portion sizes in check to avoid overeating. Use measuring cups, spoons, or visual cues to gauge appropriate serving sizes of carbohydrates, proteins, and fats.

Choose Healthy Fats: Incorporate sources of healthy fats such as avocados, nuts, seeds, olive oil, and fatty fish like salmon or trout. These fats can help improve heart health and keep you feeling full and satisfied.

Stock Up on Low-Glycemic Index Foods: Choose foods with a lower glycemic index (GI), which means they have less of an impact on blood sugar levels. Examples include beans, lentils, non-starchy vegetables, and most fruits.

Stay Hydrated: Don't forget to include beverages in your shopping list. Opt for water, herbal teas, or unsweetened beverages like sparkling water or flavored water without added sugars.

Batch Cooking and Freezing Guidelines

Batch cooking and freezing meals in advance can be a convenient strategy for managing diabetes while ensuring nutritious meals are readily available. Here are some guidelines to help you effectively batch cook and freeze diabetes-friendly meals:

Plan Your Meals: Before you start batch cooking, plan out your meals for the week. Consider recipes that are balanced with lean proteins, healthy fats, and complex carbohydrates to help regulate blood sugar levels.

Choose Diabetes-Friendly Recipes: Select recipes that use wholesome ingredients such as lean proteins (chicken, fish, tofu), non-starchy vegetables, whole grains, and legumes. Avoid recipes with excessive added sugars, refined carbohydrates, and unhealthy fats.

Invest in Quality Containers: Use high-quality, freezer-safe containers or meal prep containers to store your batch-cooked meals. Ensure they are airtight to prevent freezer burn and maintain the freshness of your food.

Label and Date Containers: Properly label each container with the name of the dish and the date it was prepared. This helps you keep track of what's in your freezer and ensures you use meals before they expire.

Cool Foods Before Freezing: Allow batch-cooked foods to cool to room temperature before placing them in the freezer. Rapid cooling helps prevent the growth of harmful bacteria and maintains the quality of the food.

Divide Meals into Portions: Divide batch-cooked meals into individual or family-sized portions before freezing. This allows for easier thawing and portion control when reheating.

Use Freezer-Friendly Ingredients: Certain ingredients freeze better than others. For example, soups, stews, casseroles, and cooked grains freeze well, while ingredients like lettuce, cucumbers, and dairy-based sauces may not retain their texture after freezing

Properly Wrap Foods: Wrap foods tightly in freezer-safe plastic wrap, aluminum foil, or freezer bags to prevent freezer burn and maintain freshness. Remove as much air as possible to minimize ice crystals.

Follow Safe Thawing Practices: Thaw frozen meals safely in the refrigerator overnight or use the defrost setting on your microwave. Avoid thawing foods at room temperature to prevent bacterial growth.

Reheat Safely: When reheating frozen meals, ensure they reach an internal temperature of 165°F (74°C) to kill any harmful bacteria. Use a food thermometer to check the temperature of the food before consuming.

CONCLUSION:

As we journey through the pages of the "Super Easy Diabetic Diet Cookbook After 50," we embark on more than just a culinary adventure. This book is a beacon of hope, a roadmap to a healthier tomorrow for those living life after 50 with diabetes. With each recipe, each ingredient carefully chosen, we're not just nourishing our bodies; we're feeding our souls with the promise of vitality and wellness.

Let's reflect on what we've discovered. We've learned that healthy eating doesn't have to be complicated. In fact, it can be downright delicious. From savory soups to tantalizing desserts, every dish in this cookbook is a celebration of flavor and nourishment.

But this journey is about more than just food. It's about empowerment. It's about taking control of our health and embracing a lifestyle that supports our well-being. It's about realizing that small changes can lead to significant transformations.

So, as we close the pages of this cookbook, let's not bid farewell to newfound knowledge and inspiration. Instead, let's carry it with us into the kitchen and beyond. Let's savor each meal, knowing that we're nourishing our bodies and nurturing our spirits.

To everyone embarking on this journey, remember: you're not alone. Together, we're a community of warriors, champions of health and vitality. Let's continue to support and uplift one another as we embrace a flavorful and balanced lifestyle, one delicious recipe at a time.

14 Days Meal Plan

Day 1:

Breakfast: Greek Yogurt with Chia Seeds and Berries

Lunch: Tofu Teriyaki with Brown Rice and Steamed Vegetables

Dinner: Baked Sweet Potato Wedges with Roasted Asparagus with Parmesan Cheese

Day 2:

Breakfast: Spiced Apple Cider (Warm Drink)

Lunch: Chicken Stir-Fry with Snow Peas, Carrots, and Cashews

Dinner: Grilled Zucchini with Lemon and Olive Oil

Day 3:

Breakfast: Breakfast Burrito

Lunch: Black Bean and Corn Quesadillas with Avocado Salsa

Dinner: Chicken Breast with Caprese Salad and Whole-Wheat Couscous

Day 4:

Breakfast: Sugar-Free Coffee with Cinnamon

Lunch: White Bean Soup with Kale and Whole-Wheat Toast

Dinner: Flank Steak Fajitas with Whole-Wheat Tortillas and Grilled Peppers

Day 5:

Breakfast: Cinnamon-Baked Apples with Walnuts

Lunch: Vegetarian Chili with Butternut Squash and Black Beans

Dinner: Baked Tofu with Peanut Sauce and Stir-Fried Vegetables

Day 6:

Breakfast: Iced Green Tea with Lemon

Lunch: Tomato and Basil Cooler

Dinner: Turkey Chili with Kidney Beans and Brown Rice

Day 7:

Breakfast: Sparkling Water with Berries and Mint

Lunch: Greek Salad with Chicken Souvlaki and Whole-Wheat Pita Bread

Dinner: Roasted Figs with Goat Cheese

Day 8:

Breakfast: Sugar-Free Hot Chocolate

Lunch: Marinated Artichoke Hearts with Coleslaw with Lightened Dressing

Dinner: Poached Pears with Spices

Day 9:

Breakfast: Homemade Fruit Salad with a Squeeze of Lemon

Lunch: Sauteed Green Beans with Garlic and Herbs

Dinner: Quinoa Salad with Chopped Vegetables and Vinaigrette

Day 10:

Breakfast: Greek Yogurt Parfait with Sliced Almonds and Berries

Lunch: Creamy Cauliflower Mash with Parmesan Cheese

Dinner: Grilled Chicken Breast with Lemon and Olive Oil

Day 11:

Breakfast: Apple Slices with Almond Butter

Lunch: Hard-boiled Eggs with Edamame Pods

Dinner: Grilled Salmon with Lemon and Dill

Day 12:

Breakfast: Berry Bliss with Chia Seed Pudding

Lunch: Sliced Turkey Breast with Whole-Wheat Crackers

Dinner: Sauteed Mushrooms with Onions and Thyme

Day 13:

Breakfast: Homemade Vegetable Juice

Lunch: Spiced Pear with Ricotta Cheese

Dinner: Baked Chicken Thighs with Garlic and Herbs

Day 14:

Breakfast: Sparkling Cranberry Limeade

Lunch: Air-Popped Popcorn with Herbs and Spices

Dinner: Coleslaw with Lightened Dressing with Marinated Artichoke Hearts

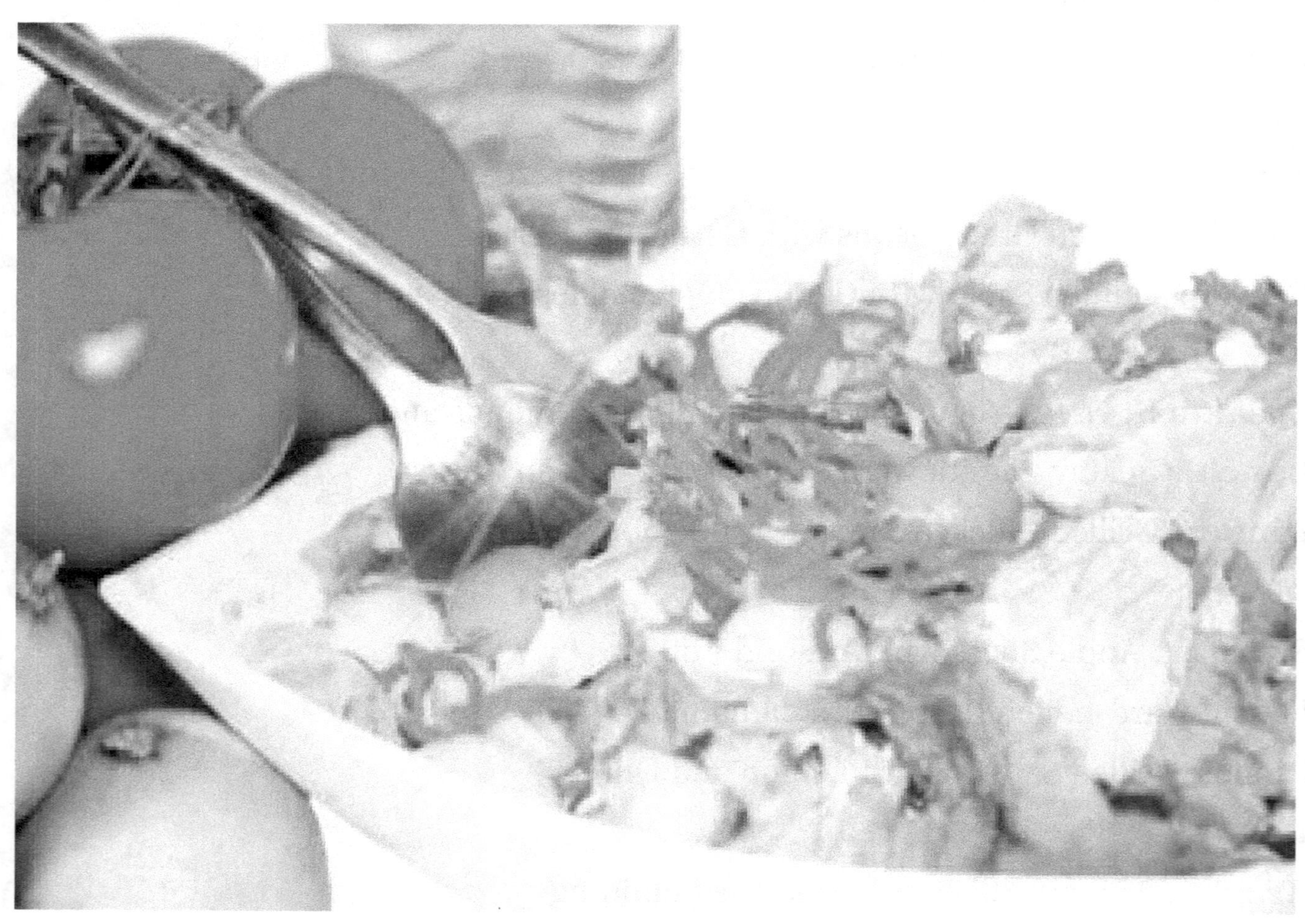